# MENISCUS LESIONS

## PRACTICAL PROBLEMS OF CLINICAL DIAGNOSIS, ARTHROGRAPHY AND THERAPY

BY

**Prof. Dr. P. RICKLIN**
MÄNNEDORF – ZURICH

**Priv.-Doz. Dr. A. RÜTTIMANN**
ZURICH

**Priv.-Doz. Dr. M.S. DEL BUONO**
ZURICH

WITH PREFACES BY

Prof. Dr. F. LANG
LUCERNE – ZURICH

Prof. Dr. H.R. SCHINZ
ZURICH

American Translation by
**KARL H. MUELLER, M.D.**
Milwaukee, Wisconsin

WITH 219 ILLUSTRATIONS

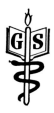

**GRUNE & STRATTON**

*A Subsidiary of Harcourt Brace Jovanovich, Publishers*

New York    San Francisco    London

*The Authors*

DEL BUONO, MANFREDI SUEVO, Privatdozent Dr. †

RICKLIN, PETER, Prof. Dr., Head of the Surgical and Gynecologic
Department of the Kreisspital Männedorf Zurich

RÜTTIMANN, ALOIS, Privatdozent Dr., Roentgen Diagnostic Central
Institute, Stadtspital Triemli, Zurich


*The Translator*

MUELLER, KARL H., M.D., Associate Professor of Orthopedic Surgery,
Marquette School of Medicine, Inc., Milwaukee, Wisconsin

Grune & Stratton, Inc., 111 Fifth Avenue, New York, N.Y. 10003

Library of Congress Catalog Card Number 76–119549

International Standard Book Number 0–8089–0652–6

Printed in West Germany (Th-B)

This book is a translation of *Die Meniscuslaesion*

© Georg Thieme Verlag, Stuttgart 1964

# Prefaces

The menisci of the knee joint are of interest not only to physicians but also to insurance companies, the courts and even to the lawmaker. Biologic and pathophysiologic changes occur in the menisci in connection with aging and natural wear and tear, trauma, increased stress from work or sports. This makes the involvement of different specialties such as roentgenology, surgery, sports medicine, preventive medicine, pathology and traumatology necessary. This monograph was written by three experienced authors, and tries to deal with all aspects of the condition: pathogenesis, including the latest developments in this field; clinical diagnosis, which is still the basis of a thorough evaluation; and the latest roentgen diagnostic procedures. Treatment, after-care and finally disability evaluation are also covered expertly.

Lucerne, January 1964          F. LANG

Evaluation of physical disorders by x-ray is often extremely important for an exact diagnosis. It can either confirm or disagree with our clinical impression and frequently clarifies the anatomical situation. X-ray examination can be important for the differential diagnosis and can also reveal significant concomitant conditions. We use it for follow-up examination of our therapeutic and especially our operative results. Diagnostic radiology plays an important role in the examination and evaluation of meniscus lesions which can be very disabling to the patient and pose difficult problems for insurance carriers. Two of my students of radiology and a surgeon have worked together to produce this excellent monograph, for which they have used their own improved modification of double contrast arthrography. This monograph is a fitting monument to our friend Del Buono, who lost his life in a tragic traffic accident.

My best wishes for success accompany this instructive monograph, which should be a valuable text for the practicing physician and the surgeon. I hope that it will be used to the benefit of all patients with meniscus and knee conditions to shorten their period of pain and disability.

Zurich, January 1964          HANS R. SCHINZ

# Foreword

The subject of meniscus lesions continues to be of great interest. Approximately every fifth meniscus injury fails to produce clear-cut symptoms. The diagnosis becomes problematic. Opinions regarding indications and technic for surgical treatment also differ widely.

We feel that a monograph written jointly by surgeons and radiologists should be of great value for the practical problems of diagnosis, treatment and evaluation of a meniscus lesion. It is our opinion that the diagnosis should be established by cooperation between radiologist and surgeon. We hope that this book will help the interested reader in the solution of the many problems posed by the injured or diseased meniscus.

We deeply regret the untimely death of our co-worker Dr. M. S. Del Buono who lost his life in a tragic traffic accident before this book was published. Dr. Del Buono came from Bari (Italy). During the last ten years, he worked as Assistant and Assistant Chief at the Central Institute for Roentgen Diagnosis of the University of Zurich and had shown great scientific potential. We have lost an excellent co-worker and a very dear friend.

We would like to take this opportunity to thank Professor Dr. F. Lang, Chairman of Accident Medicine at the University of Zurich and Director of the Swiss Accident Insurance Institute, Lucerne, as well as his County physicians for permission to use their medical charts and accident records.

We are grateful to Professor Dr. H. R. Schinz, Director of the Central Institute for X-ray Diagnosis at the University of Zurich for his generous help and the permission to use the case material of the institute.

We have received many interesting cases and good cooperation from the physicians of the Surgical Clinic of the University of Zurich under the direction of Professor Dr. A. Brunner, the Surgical Clinic-B of the University under the direction of Professor Dr. H. U. Buff and the Department of Surgery of the City Hospital of Zurich (Director: Dr. E. Kaiser) and many other colleagues in the Zurich area. We gratefully acknowledge the generous help given by Professor Dr. J. Wellauer and Professor Dr. U. Cocchi. Drs. W. Bessler, M. Grosjean, M. Maranta and W. Fuchs and many other physicians of the Central Institute for Roentgen Diagnosis of the University of Zurich have helped us with the arthrograms. Dr. Charlotte Fuchs-Schmid, Mr. Jacques Keller and Mr. Ivan Glitsch have made the photocopies and drawings. To Sister Hulda Abderhalden and many other co-workers in the Central Institute for Roentgen Diagnosis, we owe a debt of gratitude.

Our special thanks go to Mr. Günther Hauff and his co-workers of the Georg Thieme Verlag for their excellent job in printing and producing this book.

Männedorf and Zurich, January 1964

PETER RICKLIN
ALOIS RÜTTIMANN

# Table of Contents

Prefaces . . . . . . . . . . . . . . . . . . . . . . . . . . . . . . . . . . . . . . . . iii

Foreword . . . . . . . . . . . . . . . . . . . . . . . . . . . . . . . . . . . . . . . . . v

Introduction . . . . . . . . . . . . . . . . . . . . . . . . . . . . . . . . . . . . . . . . 1

CHAPTER 1

**Anatomical and Physiological Considerations** . . . . . . . . . . . . . . . . . . . . . . 2

1) Anatomy of the Knee Joint . . . . . . . 2    2) Mechanics of Movement of the Knee Joint   6

CHAPTER 2

**Pathogenesis of Meniscus Lesions** . . . . . . . . . . . . . . . . . . . . . . . . . . . . 7

1) Mechanical Causes . . . . . . . . . . . 7    c) Degenerative Changes . . . . . . . . 10

2) Factors Which Increase Vulnerability . . . 9    d) Specific Activities . . . . . . . . . . 10

   a) Constitutional and Congenital Variations   9    3) Typical Lesions . . . . . . . . . . . . 13

   b) Ligamentous Damage . . . . . . . . 9    4) Classification of Meniscus Lesions . . . . 14

CHAPTER 3

**Clinical Diagnosis** . . . . . . . . . . . . . . . . . . . . . . . . . . . . . . . . . . . . 16

1) History . . . . . . . . . . . . . . . 16    c) Böhler's Sign . . . . . . . . . . . 21

2) Initial Symptoms . . . . . . . . . . . 17    d) Payr's Sign . . . . . . . . . . . . 21

3) Locking . . . . . . . . . . . . . . . 17    e) 1st Steinmann's Sign . . . . . . . . 21

4) Clinical Examination . . . . . . . . . 18    f) Merke's Sign . . . . . . . . . . . 21

5) Meniscus Signs . . . . . . . . . . . . 20    g) McMurray Test . . . . . . . . . . 22

   a) 2nd Steinmann's Sign . . . . . . . . 20    h) Apley Test . . . . . . . . . . . . 22

   b) Bragard's Sign . . . . . . . . . . 20

CHAPTER 4

**Routine X-Ray Examination of the Knee** . . . . . . . . . . . . . . . . . . . . . . . . . 23

CHAPTER 5

**Arthrography** . . . . . . . . . . . . . . . . . . . . . . . . . . . . . . . . . . . . . . . 24

A. *Historical Review* . . . . . . . . . . . 24    7) Technical Errors . . . . . . . . . . . 31

B. *Introduction and Indications* . . . . . . 25    D. *The Normal Arthrogram* . . . . . . . 31

C. *Methodology* . . . . . . . . . . . . . 25    1) The Normal Meniscus . . . . . . . . . 31

1) Materials . . . . . . . . . . . . . . 25    a) Variations in the Normal Arthrogram of

2) Contrast Media . . . . . . . . . . . 26     the Medial Meniscus . . . . . . . . 36

3) Technic . . . . . . . . . . . . . . . 26    b) Variations of the Normal Lateral Menis-

   a) Puncture of the Joint . . . . . . . . 26     cus . . . . . . . . . . . . . . . . 44

   b) Evacuation of Joint Effusion . . . . . 27    2) Joint Spaces and Joint Capsule . . . . . 45

   c) Injection of Contrast Media . . . . . 27    3) Bursae . . . . . . . . . . . . . . . 47

4) Equipment . . . . . . . . . . . . . 28    4) The Infrapatellar Fat Pad . . . . . . . 50

5) Physical Basis for Meniscus Visualization . 28    5) The Dorsal Fat Pad . . . . . . . . . 50

6) X-Ray Technic . . . . . . . . . . . . 29    6) The Cruciate Ligaments . . . . . . . . 50

   a) Visualization of the Medial Meniscus . . 29    7) Articular Surfaces . . . . . . . . . . 52

   b) Visualization of the Lateral Meniscus . . 30    8) Anatomical Characteristics of Different Me-

   c) Multiple Views . . . . . . . . . . 30     niscus Segments in Serial Views . . . . . 52

   d) Visualization of Other Intra-articular    E. *The Abnormal Arthrogram* . . . . . . . 53

    Structures . . . . . . . . . . . . . 31    1) Meniscus Injuries . . . . . . . . . . 53

a) Longitudinal Tears. . . . . . . . . .     55
b) Transverse Tears . . . . . . . . . .     56
c) Complex Tears (Mixed Forms). . . . .     57
d) Complete Detachment (Disinsertion) . .     57
2) Degenerative Meniscus Changes . . . . .     71
3) Developmental Anomalies of the Menisci .     75
F. Status Post-Meniscectomy . . . . . . .     75
G. Sources of Diagnostic Errors . . . . . .     78
1) Errors in Technic . . . . . . . . . .     82
a) Periarticular Injection of Contrast Medium. . . . . . . . . . . . . . .     82
b) Incomplete Evacuation of Joint Effusions     85
2) Errors in X-Ray Technic . . . . . . .     85
a) Projection Not Orthograde . . . . . .     85
b) Excessive Rotation . . . . . . . .     85

3) Errors in the Anatomical Differentiation of
the Arthrogram . . . . . . . . . . .     85
a) Superimposition of the Infrapatellar Fat
Pad . . . . . . . . . . . . . . .     85
b) Superimposition of the Recessus . . . .     86
c) Superimposition of a Bursa . . . . . .     88
d) Connection of the Posterior Horn of the
Medial Meniscus with the Capsule . . .     89
e) The Popliteal Hiatus. . . . . . . . .     89
f) Our Own Errors. . . . . . . . . . .     89
H. Complications of Double Contrast Arthrography . . . . . . . . . . . . . . .     90
I. Radiation Exposure . . . . . . . . . .     93
1) Exposure of the Patient. . . . . . . .     93
2) Radiation Exposure of the Examiner . . .     93

CHAPTER 6

## Clinical and Radiologic Differential Diagnosis . . . . . . . . . . . . . . . . . . . .     93

1) Ligamentous and Capsular Damage. . . .     93
a) Collateral Ligament and Capsule Lesions     93
b) Lesions of the Cruciate Ligaments . . .     96
2) Cartilage and Bone Changes . . . . . .     98
a) Arthrosis Deformans . . . . . . . . .     98
b) Osteochondritis Dissecans. . . . . . .     99
c) Osteochondromatosis. . . . . . . . .     103
d) Chondromalacia Patellae . . . . . . .     104
3) Synovitis and Bursitis . . . . . . . . .     105

a) Chronic Synovitis . . . . . . . . . .     105
b) Hoffa's Disease . . . . . . . . . . .     106
c) Villous Synovitis . . . . . . . . . .     107
d) Diseases of the Bursae . . . . . . . .     107
4) Ganglia and Tumors . . . . . . . . . .     107
a) Ganglia of the Menisci . . . . . . . .     107
b) Ganglia of the Capsule . . . . . . . .     110
c) Tumors of the Knee Joint . . . . . .     110

CHAPTER 7

## Therapeutic Problems . . . . . . . . . . . . . . . . . . . . . . . . . . . . . . . .     110

1) Indications for Conservative and Operative
Therapy . . . . . . . . . . . . . . .     111
a) Fresh Traumatic Tears . . . . . . . .     111
b) Late Changes Following Traumatic Tears     111
c) Spontaneous Detachment (Meniscopathy)     112
d) Late Changes in Unstable Joints. . . .     112
2) Conservative Treatment. . . . . . . . .     112
3) Operative Treatment . . . . . . . . . .     114
a) Partial or Total Meniscectomy . . . .     114
b) Instruments . . . . . . . . . . . .     116
c) Preparation for Surgery . . . . . . .     117
d) Anesthesia . . . . . . . . . . . .     117
e) Positioning and Tourniquet Control . .     118

f) Incision . . . . . . . . . . . . . .     118
g) Technic of Resection . . . . . . . . .     120
h) After-Care . . . . . . . . . . . . .     122
4) Postoperative Complications. . . . . . .     124
a) Postoperative Pain . . . . . . . . .     124
b) Infection . . . . . . . . . . . . . .     124
c) Disturbances of Wound Healing . . . .     125
d) Quadriceps Weakness . . . . . . . . .     126
e) Meniscus Remnants . . . . . . . . .     126
f) Chronic Synovitis . . . . . . . . . .     126
g) Sudeck's Dystrophy . . . . . . . . .     127
h) Arthrosis Deformans . . . . . . . . .     128

CHAPTER 8

## Disability Evaluation . . . . . . . . . . . . . . . . . . . . . . . . . . . . . . . . .     129

Bibliography. . . . . . . . . . . . . . .     133     Index . . . . . . . . . . . . . . . . . . . .     139

# Introduction

With increasing development of subspecialties, cooperation of the different specialists in the treatment of patients becomes more and more important. This book was born from such teamwork. It is of interest both to the surgeon and the radiologist and deals primarily with the practical aspects of diagnosis and treatment of the most important internal derangement of the knee joint – the damaged meniscus.

The increased incidence of knee injuries in sports and industry has produced continuous improvement of diagnostic facilities. In most cases the experienced examiner will be able to diagnose a meniscus lesion with sufficient certainty from the history and a thorough clinical examination. Clinical diagnosis, however, has its limitations because there are meniscus lesions without typical signs and symptoms. Statistical analysis of the accuracy of different meniscus symptoms and signs shows all of them to have a certain percentage of errors. Schaer has shown that diagnostic difficulties are to be expected in approximately 15 per cent of all cases. Exploratory arthrotomy is not a satisfactory solution to the problem because it carries a certain risk and should only be considered as a last resort when all other measures fail.

Only 10 years ago Smillie considered the practical importance of arthrography to be small, but expressed the hope that its technic would be improved. This has been accomplished in the meantime. Lindblom in Sweden has developed arthrography with a liquid contrast medium. Van de Berg and Crevecoeur have developed the double contrast method. Many other authors have made contributions to the improvement of arthrography.

In experienced hands arthrography of the knee joint can reduce the number of diagnostic problems to a minimum. Our own error rate, like that of Lindblom, is approximately 5 per cent. Catolla, Van de Berg, and Crevecoeur have recently reported successful eliminations of false findings altogether. Exact knowledge and experience in the technic of arthrography, however, is an absolute prerequisite for achieving satisfactory results. This was the reason for writing a section on arthrography in textbook form. We have also dealt with the technical difficulties and the diagnostic errors which have occurred in our material of 2500 arthrographies and 600 operative cases. The reader can obtain a certain amount of diagnostic accuracy by thorough study of this chapter. We hope that this will help the inexperienced to avoid some of the early difficulties. According to its practical importance we have also dealt more extensively with the differential diagnosis of meniscus injuries and have given both clinical symptomatology and radiographic diagnosis the necessary consideration.

A multiplicity of problems has to be dealt with in the treatment of meniscus lesions. Although meniscectomy is a routine operation in every major clinic today, opinions about the most suitable approach vary considerably. We have described our own operative technic which has proven itself over many years. We realize, however, that satisfactory results can be obtained with other methods.

Since every meniscus lesion raises the question of a possible traumatic origin, we have also discussed some of the problems of disability evaluation.

# CHAPTER 1

# Anatomical and Physiological Considerations

## 1) Anatomy of the Knee Joint

Thorough knowledge of anatomy and function of the knee joint is a prerequisite for the understanding of the mechanism of meniscus injuries, for diagnostic evaluation of knee complaints, for the technic and evaluation of knee arthrograms and especially for the successful excision of damaged menisci.

The knee joint is the most complicated joint of the human body. It is formed by the distal end of the femur and the proximal epiphysis of the tibia which are joined by several important structures to form a stable and statically safe joint (Toendury). The osseous and soft tissue structures are arranged in a manner to permit minimal rotational movements in addition to extension and flexion. Abduction and adduction also are made possible to a certain degree with widening of the medial or lateral joint space.

The articular surface of the *femur* has a patellar and a tibial surface (Figs. 1 and 2). The patellar surface is a flat asymmetrical saddle, the lateral part of which is larger than the medial. Both femoral condyles correspond to the two articular condyles of the tibia. The medial femoral condyle has a smaller transverse and a larger longitudinal diameter than the lateral condyle. The lateral femoral condyle occasionally shows a small transverse groove in the center of its cartilage-covered surface.

The *tibial plateau* has two articular surfaces. The medial surface is oval-shaped in a dorso-

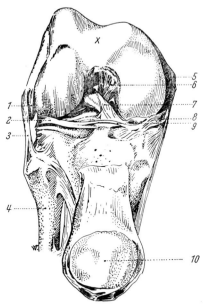

Fig. 1. Front view of the right knee joint. x = Facies patellaris of the articular surface of the femur. 1. Tendon sheath of the popliteus tendon. 2. Lateral meniscus. 3. Lateral collateral ligament. 4. Fibula. 5. Joint capsule. 6. Posterior cruciate ligament. 7. Anterior cruciate ligament. 8. Medial meniscus. 9. Transverse ligament. 10. Articular surface of the patella.

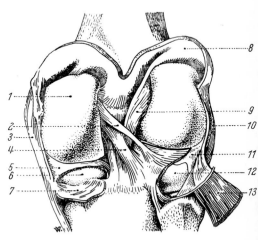

Fig. 2. Posterior view of the right knee joint. 1. Medial femoral condyle. 2. Ligamentum menisci fibularis. 3. Medial collateral ligament. 4. Posterior cruciate ligament. 5. Medial meniscus. 6. Posterior aspect of the medial tibial plateau. 7. Posterior capsule. 8. Joint capsule. 9. Anterior cruciate ligament. 10. Lateral collateral ligament. 11. Lateral meniscus. 12. Bursa musculi poplitei. 13. Popliteus muscle.

ventral direction and is more concave. The lateral surface is smaller and has a more round configuration.

The two articular surfaces of the tibia are angulated slightly towards each other and are separated by the eminentia intercondylaris, which has a medial and a lateral spine. As an occasional variant a third spur can be present as the tuberculum tertium on the ventral side and the tuberculum quartum on the dorsal side. The *articular cartilage* in the adult has an average thickness of 3 to 4 mm.

The dorsal aspect of the *patella* is covered with cartilage. This articular surface forms a flattened roof with a ridge in the vertical direction. The lateral portion of the patella is larger and more concave than the medial surface.

The *joint capsule* is large and shallow, especially in its anterior portion. This makes it possible to inject considerable amounts of air (approximately 40 cc.) into the joint without tension. The joint capsule is reinforced by the medial collateral ligament which is incorporated into the capsule by the ligamentum popliteum obliquum and arcuatum in the popliteal area, whereas the lateral collateral ligament has no connection with the joint capsule. The capsule inserts into the femur near the border of the cartilaginous articular surface at the junction of the epicondyles and condyles. The joint capsule inserts into the tibia just distal to the collateral ligaments. The semimembranosus muscle tightens the capsule on its relatively short dorsal side. The incongruence of the articulating surfaces of femur and tibia is equalized to a certain degree by the *menisci*. These are wedge-shaped fibrocartilaginous structures which are located on the periphery of the articular surface of the tibia, and are connected with the joint capsule.

These menisci are the rudiments of an embryonic septum between tibia and fibula. They have a semilunar form, their cross-section is wedge-shaped with the apex of the wedge directed towards the interior of the joint.

The menisci are mobile buffers which distribute the pressure of the femur over a larger area of the tibia and increase the elasticity of the joint (Toendury). Menisci and ligaments of this joint form a functional unit. Each meniscus has

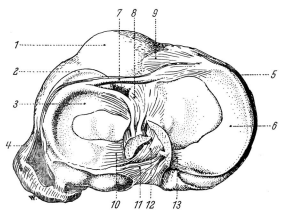

Fig. 3. Articular surface of the left tibia with menisci seen from above. 1. Tuberositas tibiae. 2. Anterior aspect of the articular portion of the lateral tibial plateau. 3. Lateral meniscus, anterior horn. 4. Tibiofibular ligament. 5. Medial tibial plateau. 6. Medial meniscus, middle portion. 7. Transverse ligament. 8. Attachment of the anterior cruciate ligament. 9. Ligamentous attachment of the anterior horn of the medial meniscus to the tibia. 10. Posterior attachment of the lateral meniscus. 11. Ligamentum menisci fibularis. 12. Posterior cruciate ligament. 13. Posterior attachment of the medial meniscus.

an osseous insertion in the area intercondylaris anterior and posterior. The insertions of the medial meniscus surround those of the lateral meniscus (Fig. 3).

The average width of the *medial meniscus* is approximately 10 mm. with its posterior horn usually a little wider than the middle and anterior portions. The medial meniscus has a wider curve than the lateral meniscus and follows the periphery of the medial tibial plateau.

The anterior horn has a ligamentous connection with the anterior ridge of the tibia and the ventral ridge of the eminentia intercondylaris. It frequently has a connection with the anterior cruciate ligament. The ligamentum transversum connects it ventrally with the lateral meniscus. The mobility of the medial meniscus is limited by its tight connection with the joint capsule and the medial collateral ligament. This makes the medial meniscus more prone to injuries than the lateral meniscus. The connection between the medial meniscus and the capsule posteriorly is occasionally lengthened by a short bridge of tissue.

The average width of the *lateral meniscus* measures 12 to 13 mm. which is considerably more than that of the medial meniscus. Its curvature is much smaller and its appearance is almost that of a closed ring. Variants of form are much more frequent in the lateral meniscus than in the medial meniscus and are secondary to developmental disturbances which will be discussed in more detail below.

The anterior and posterior horns of the lateral meniscus insert directly into the eminentia intercondylaris. The ligamentum menisci fibularis connects the posterior horn with the posterior cruciate ligament. The major portion of the posterior horn inserts directly into the femur in the fossa intercondylaris. The lateral meniscus has only loose connections with the joint capsule. On the ventral side these are usually thin wedges of tissue. In the area of the posterior horn connections with the joint capsule are interrupted by the tendon sheath of the popliteal tendon

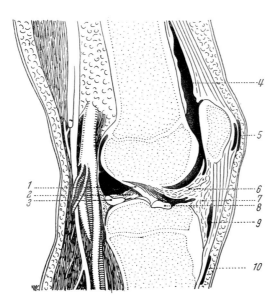

Fig. 4. Sagittal section through the knee joint (after Töndury). 1. Anterior cruciate ligament. 2. Posterior cruciate ligament. 3. Section through the posterior horn of the lateral meniscus. 4. Superior recessus. 5. Subcutaneous pre-patellar bursa. 6 and 7. Fat pad with infrapatellar synovial fold. 8. Section through the anterior horn of the lateral meniscus. 9. Deep infrapatellar bursa. 10. Subcutaneous infrapatellar bursa.

(Fig. 2). This area is located immediately posterior to the lateral collateral ligament. According to Heim this portion of the lateral meniscus measures approximately 2 to 4 cm. Dorsal-lateral to the tibial plateau we also find a synovial pocket of equal distance between meniscus and capsule which is called recessus inferior. This recessus is wide open proximally and becomes smaller distally. Its outside wall contains the tendon of the popliteal muscle which forms a cord-like bulge in the wall. The recessus or synovial pocket has been called the sheath of the popliteal tendon (Spalteholz) or bursa musculi poplitei. Occasionally the tendon of the popliteal muscle lies completely free between the meniscus and the capsule. (See Figs. 56 and 57.)

Between the undersurface of the lateral meniscus and the recessus we often find an open connection of approximately 1 to 2 cm. width. It is bounded on both sides by a sail-like ligament which anchors the meniscus to the posterior surface of the tibia (Heim, Wieser). The cranial border of the lateral meniscus is fixed to the joint capsule by another sail-like ligament which blends into the medial muscle fibers of the popliteus (Last). Since its bony insertions are located closer together and no tight connections with the collateral ligament exist, the lateral meniscus has considerably more mobility than the medial.

*Vascular Supply*

The popliteal artery has five branches in the area of the knee joint. The two proximal branches form the so-called rete articulare genus in the capsule and do not supply the meniscus. These are followed by the arteria genus media and more distally by the paired arteriae genus distales.

The arteria genus media perforates the joint capsule posteriorly and divides into three main branches: a central branch which follows the posterior cruciate ligament, a medial branch which goes horizontally into the parameniscal zone medially, and a lateral branch which supplies the parameniscal zone laterally in the same manner.

The arteriae genus distales consist of one medial and one lateral branch which perforate the joint capsule, run ventrally, and join to form an arch under the ligamentum patellae. From there they send out branches to the parameniscal areas bilaterally.

The parameniscal zone consists of loose connective tissue and either contains a single larger artery or several smaller arteries which supply the surrounding tissue. These arteries go only into the outer one-third of the meniscus. The menisci are vascularized only in their peripheral zone which is contrasted sharply to the inner avascular parts (Fig. 5).

The anterior and the posterior horns are somewhat less vascularized than the central portions of the medial menisci. The lateral meniscus has a better vascular supply than the medial.

Histologically the vascular supply of the meniscus is not uniform. The smallest vessels run from the periphery into the outer portion of the meniscus in a tongue-shaped fashion and vary in caliber. Anastomoses are rare in this zone. (Bombeli, Luna). Histologically even the outer one-third of the meniscus shows areas which are avascular.

The capillaries do not form a net but are arranged in a coil-like manner to facilitate shifting. The vascular supply to the surface of the meniscus is less than that to the deeper portions of the tissue.

Histologically the meniscus can be divided into three zones (Fig. 5):

1) A cartilaginous avascular zone which contains the inner three-fourths of the meniscus.
2) A fibrous zone which contains capillaries.
3) A parameniscal zone consisting of loose connective tissue.

The fibrous zone merges smoothly with the parameniscal zone. The latter corresponds to the vascular connection between capsule and meniscus.

Besides the lateral ligaments the *cruciate ligaments* contribute considerably to the stability of the knee joint (Figs. 3 and 4). The anterior cruciate ligament arises from the inner side of the lateral femoral condyle and inserts into the anterior part of the eminentia intercondylaris. By its oblique course it limits mainly the anterior displacement of the tibia against the femur (anterior drawer sign). The posterior cruciate liga-

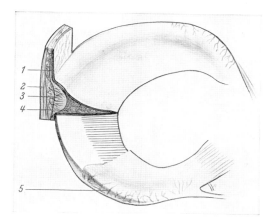

Fig. 5. Anatomic cross-section through the meniscus. 1. Stratum superficiale. 2. Joint capsule. 3. Premeniscal vascular zone of regeneration. 4. Avascular hyaline cartilage. 5. Vessels of the zone of regeneration.

ment arises from the medial femoral condyle in the fossa intercondylaris, and inserts into the dorsal surface of the eminentia intercondylaris. It prevents posterior displacement of the tibia. Both cruciate ligaments limit external rotation of the femur on the fixed tibia and also prevent abnormal internal rotation of the tibia on the femur. The synovial membrane of the joint capsule covers the cruciate ligaments from the dorsal side which gives the ligaments extra-articular location.

The knee joint can be divided into several compartments (Fig. 4).

The *anterior compartment* continues cranially into the recessus anterior superior (bursa suprapatellaris). The latter is frequently separated by an incomplete and rarely by a complete septum. (See Fig. 62.)

The *anterior infrapatellar fat pad* narrows the anterior compartment below the patella. The fat pad is adherent to the joint capsule which is reinforced by the ligamentum patellae. The *posterior fat pad*, which lies behind the cruciate ligaments, divides the *posterior compartment* into two parts vertically. The posterior and anterior compartments are divided into a superior and inferior capsular space by the menisci.

Several of the *bursae* can have connections with the joint space, mainly the bursa poplitea

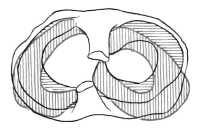

Fig. 6. Position of the menisci with the knee in extension (black) and flexion (red) (after Schaer).

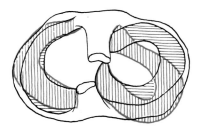

Fig. 7. Position of the menisci with the knee in extension (black), and flexion with internal rotation of the tibia (red) (after Schaer).

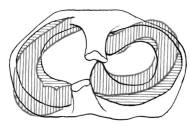

Fig. 8. Position of the menisci with the knee in extension (black) and flexion with external rotation of the tibia (red) (after Schaer).

through the tendon sheath of the popliteal muscle, the bursa semimembranosogastrocnemia and several smaller accessory bursae.

## 2) Mechanics of Movement of the Knee Joint

The knee joint is a hinge joint which also allows rotatory movements to a limited degree.

In extension the joint is fixed rigidly by its capsular and ligamentous structures. Flexion beyond 20 degrees relaxes the collateral and cruciate ligaments because the femoral condyles decrease in size posteriorly. Relaxation of the lateral collateral ligaments is more marked then that of the medial collateral ligament. Some instability of the knee joint laterally and medially in incomplete extension is physiologic. Displacement of the tibia against the femur of several millimeters in the saggital plane is not a pathologic finding.

The increasing relaxation of the ligamentous structures when the knee is flexed also allows rotatory movements by gliding displacement of the femoral condyles on the tibial plateau. Since the axis of rotation does not go through the center of the joint, but through the medial condyle of the tibia, the lateral femoral condyle displaces more than the medial femoral condyle.

The rotatory motion which takes place in the end phase of extension or in the beginning of flexion, respectively, is of special importance. Due to its slightly flattened shape, the medial femoral condyle displaces posteriorly during the last 20 degrees of extension when the tibia is fixed. This screwing motion in the form of an internal rotation locks the joint securely. By the same token the femur rotates externally during the first 20 degrees of flexion.

Flexion causes the *menisci* to slide posteriorly on the tibial plateau. Because of its tight fixation to the joint capsule, the medial meniscus displaces considerably less than the lateral meniscus (Fig. 6). With extreme flexion the posterior horn of the medial meniscus is compressed between femur and tibia and can be damaged easily.

When rotatory motion is added to flexion of the knee, displacement of the lateral meniscus is even more pronounced. (Figs. 7 and 8 show the position of the menisci in internal and external rotation of the tibia.) Extreme movements can cause the menisci to protrude over the articular surface of the tibia.

External rotation of the tibia is always possible to a greater degree than internal rotation, which is checked by the cruciate ligaments. Flexion and extension take place mainly between the femur and the menisci, while rotatory movements occur predominantly between the menisci and the tibia.

Stability of the knee joint depends on the ligamentous structures, but also to a considerable degree on the tone of the musculature acting upon the knee joint. Most significant of these is the quadriceps muscle and its important component, the vastus medialis. The latter exerts its main effectiveness in the last 10 to 15 degrees of extension and is responsible for the "screwing home" motion and stability of the joint in extension. Of lesser importance are the gastroc- nemius, the popliteus, and the iliotibial tract. The importance of the musculature, and especially that of the quadriceps, can become apparent in the presence of ligamentous damage to the knee joint, which can be compensated to a considerable degree by well-developed extensor muscles.

CHAPTER 2

# Pathogenesis of Meniscus Lesions

The causes which can lead to damage or injury to the menisci are multiple. Many factors play a role and reconstruction of the exact mechanism of injury which produced the lesion is impossible in many cases. This is one of the main reasons for the difficulties which can arise in the evaluation of disability due to a meniscus lesion.

We know that the medial meniscus is damaged much more frequently than the lateral. There are, however, considerable regional variations which correspond to the different injuries in work and sports. In athletic injuries the ratio of medial meniscus lesions to those of the lateral meniscus is 3 to 1 (Groh, Smillie); in miners we find a ratio which can go as high as 20 to 1 (Andreesen, Buerkle de la Camp). In a mixed series the average ratio is approximately 8 to 1 (Breitenfelder, Bossard, Jakoby, Krömer, Remen, Ritzmann, and others).

The greater incidence of medial meniscus lesions emphasize the fact that in addition to purely anatomical reasons, meniscus lesions are caused first of all by mechanical factors. These problems will be discussed in the following chapter.

## 1) Mechanical Causes

Damage or tear of a meniscus usually occurs when the cartilage is exposed to abnormal pressure or tension. This occurs when the weight-bearing joint is subjected to a combined flexion-rotation or extension-rotation motion.

The intact knee joint is fixed securely in full extension; therefore, lateral displacement and rotatory movements are impossible. Injuries to the menisci in full extension are possible only when ligamentous damage or a fracture of the tibial plateau occur at the same time.

The elastic fibrous structure of the menisci, the rigid fixation of the anterior and posterior horns and their connections with the joint capsule cause the menisci to return to their normal position at the periphery of the joint after each displacement. Disturbance of the normal mechanism of the joint and interference with the mobility of the menisci can exceed their elasticity and cause tears of the cartilaginous substance. This seems to occur most frequently when a meniscus which is displaced into the joint is caught between femoral and tibial condyles because of a sudden change of movement.

Based on Konjetzny's theoretical considerations, Schaer has tried to explain tears of the menisci in the following manner: The femoral and tibial condyles grasp the meniscus which is displaced into the joint like a pair of pliers, crush it, tear it longitudinally, and displace it into the joint either partially or totally (Fig. 9).

Figure 9 shows that before this can happen, the respective joint space must be opened temporarily by a valgus or varus stress. The cartilage is damaged by the sudden closure of the jaws of the bony pliers (Groh). Konjetzny related the greater incidence of medial meniscus

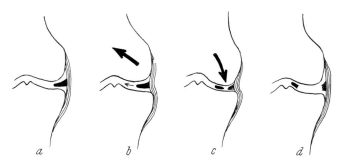

Fig. 9. Mechanism of meniscus tear (after Konjetzny and Schaer). a) Normal position. b) Flexion, external rotation and forced valgus position displaces the meniscus into the interior of the joint. c) Sudden extension crushes the meniscus between the bony condyles. d) Displacement of the detached meniscus fragment into the intercondylar notch.

injuries mainly to differences in the curvature of the articular surfaces of the tibia. In contrast to the slightly convex lateral articular surface of the tibia, the medial articular surface is somewhat concave, which favors displacement of the meniscus into the joint.

We share the opinion of Krömer, Smillie, and others that typical longitudinal tears of the medial meniscus are caused by its rigid connections with the joint capsule and the collateral ligament which create tension forces from the periphery. Internal rotation of the flexed femur on the fixed tibia displaces the medial meniscus posteriorly. This displacement is counteracted by the elasticity of the cartilaginous tissue, its connections with the joint capsule and the collateral ligament, and the bony attachments of the anterior and posterior horn. The meniscus is first drawn into the joint space where tension fixes it between the femoral and tibial condyles. Sudden extension of the joint can create considerable tension forces between the fixed meniscus and the joint capsule which will cause a tear when the tolerance of the cartilaginous tissue or the fibrous connections with the capsule and ligament are exceeded. If the tear is small, the meniscus will return to its normal position. A tear which extends into the anterior horn (bucket handle tear) can displace the free segment of the meniscus into the joint and cause typical locking. Experience has shown that a complete longitudinal tear occurs in only a small percentage of cases with this first injury. Quite frequently a partial tear will result which is then extended into the typical bucket-handle tear by repeated injuries. Smillie in his series reports approximately the same number of bucket-handle tears

resulting from one-time injuries and from multiple injuries (52 versus 48 per cent). Kroemer and others, on the other hand, believe that bucket-handle tears are usually the result of multiple injuries.

The frequent finding of early damage on the underside of the meniscus can be explained by the fact that with rotation the cartilage will move with the femoral condyle on the tibial plateau which creates abnormal forces, especially between the undersurface of the meniscus and the tibial plateau (Smillie). This mechanism of injury based on a tension effect of the capsular and ligamentous structures helps us explain the much higher incidence of injuries to the medial meniscus. The lateral meniscus, which is almost closed like a ring, has only loose connections to the joint capsule, no direct connections to the lateral collateral ligament, and a much greater mobility. The lateral meniscus can thus more easily avoid being caught by the femoral condyle, and is subjected to tension forces to a much lesser degree.

This theory, of course, does not explain all meniscus tears, and many other mechanisms of injury can be postulated. A transverse tear, for instance, can occur when excessive displacement of the meniscus stretches its concave inner border and tears it. Because of its greater curvature, transverse tears occur more frequently in the lateral meniscus. Aside from all theoretical considerations we would like to mention again, however, that the important factors for an injury to the menisci are combinations of uncontrolled flexion or extension with rotatory movements. These movements interfere with the normal mobility of the menisci and make them vulnerable to excessive tension and compression forces.

## 2) Factors Which Increase Vulnerability

### a) *Constitutional and Congenital Variations*

The fact that some people have two, sometimes three or even all four menisci removed within the course of a few years seems to indicate that *constitutional* factors can increase vulnerability of a meniscus to a certain degree. This can be due to inferior quality of cartilaginous tissue and the presence of generalized connective tissue weakness. In the presence of a weak thigh musculature and ligamentous relaxation, the connections between menisci and joint capsule are undoubtedly also lax and the menisci can easily be caught between the condyles and suffer damage (de Palma). It has also been mentioned that overweight people with poorly developed musculature are more prone to meniscus lesions than persons of normal weight and athletic build. The well-known fact that 90 per cent of all meniscus lesions are in men and only approximately 10 per cent in women indicates that specific activities in sports and work are much more important etiologically than constitutional factors.

Predisposition to meniscus lesions is also due to form and size of the menisci. In patients where both the medial or lateral menisci have to be removed, we frequently find similar or identical tears. We have already mentioned that congenital variations of form are more frequent in the lateral meniscus. It can be easily understood that abnormally wide ring-shaped and especially discoid menisci are more prone to damage than slender, narrow cartilaginous wedges.

### b) *Ligamentous Damage*

In order to withstand the many stresses placed upon it during daily living, the knee joint needs intact muscles and ligaments. These structures are absolutely necessary for correct function and stability of the knee joint. Instability of the joint from ligamentous damage or inadequate thigh musculature predisposes to internal derangement of the knee joint. Accordingly we frequently find relaxation or ruptures of the

collateral or cruciate ligaments in addition to the meniscus injuries. In late cases Groh found collateral ligament damage in 58 per cent and cruciate ligament damage in 37 per cent. These frequently occur as combined injuries at the time of the meniscus lesion. Frequently the symptomatology in a fresh knee injury is not very characteristic, or the symptoms of ligamentous injury predominate. A lesion of the

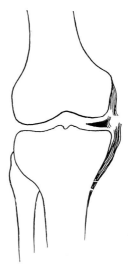

Fig. 10. Detachment of the meniscus with tear of the medial collateral ligament.

medial collateral ligament at the level of the joint line will almost always cause a partial detachment of the meniscus (Fig. 10). Krömer has pointed out that these concomitant injuries of the meniscus usually show a good tendency to heal because the injury is located in a vascular area. When treatment is inadequate, however, this can lead to a typical meniscus lesion.

Ligamentous insufficiency and especially instability of the knee can lead to late lesions of the menisci even without primary injury. Inadequate stability of the joint with its unphysiological gliding and shearing motions squeeze the cartilages between the condyles and cause them to degenerate prematurely. If at the same time weakness of the quadriceps exists, normal mechanics of the knee joint are disturbed even more. In these cases even minimal trauma, which under normal circumstances would not lead to cartilage injuries, can cause meniscus tears and locking of the knee.

### c) *Degenerative Changes*

Multiple stresses and strains act upon the skeletal system during life. Similar to the changes in the spine and the articular surfaces of the lower extremity, the cartilaginous substance of the menisci can often show its first degenerative changes in the second decade of life. We would refer here to the thorough histologic investigations of Ceelen, Ishido, Niessen, Schaer, Siegmund, Tobler, and others, who found fine droplets of lipoid in the cartilage cells and the intercellular substance. These changes are first limited to the superficial layers, but can later extend to the deep layers of the cartilage. After age 30 and even more frequently in later years, we find degenerative changes in the structure which can decrease elasticity and resistance of the menisci. The intracellular substance shows inclusions of fatty droplets, mucinous or hyaline degeneration. In addition to circumscribed necroses we occasionally find calcification of the ground substance. Macroscopically these menisci show a spotty yellow surface with small fissures and tears. Frequently the surface is fibrillated in an asbestos-like manner.

The extent of these degenerative changes varies from one individual to another. In some cases we find marked degenerative changes of the intercellular substance in the third or fourth decade; while occasionally the menisci in very old people are practically normal. The stresses and strains to which the knee joint is subjected in daily living play an important role in the etiology of these degenerative changes. It has been shown that activities which require prolonged work in a kneeling or squatting position accelerate degeneration of the menisci. Marked flexion of the knees which in a kneeling or squatting position is combined with external rotation of the tibiae causes marked dorsal displacement of the medial meniscus. This places the anterior portion of the cartilage under abnormal tension while the posterior horn is pulled

between the condyles and crushed. If these activities are carried out over a period of months and years they can lead to pressure necrosis of the menisci (Andreesen, Buerkle de la Camp). The borderlines between physiological wear and pathologic degeneration are difficult to define in most cases. This is one of the main reasons for the difficulties and uncertainties in disability evaluation of a meniscus lesion. We agree with Schaer that the situation is similar to that of arteriosclerosis of the vessels, where differentiation of the borderlines between physiologic and pathologic changes depends largely upon the decision of the examiner.

In this chapter we must also mention *ganglia* of the menisci which are localized cysts caused by mucinous or gelatinous degeneration. They are usually found in the lateral meniscus and are frequently associated with localized transverse or oblique tears. It must be assumed that the cystic degeneration, which usually involves the adjoining joint capsule, limits the meniscus in its mobility and causes it to tear more easily.

### d) *Specific Activities*

Existing evidence indicates that in the majority of cases meniscus injuries are the result of *indirect trauma*. It is theoretically possible that blunt force can occasionally crush and tear a meniscus between femur and tibia. Both menisci are, however, relatively well-protected by the protruding head of the tibia. Injury by direct force as a rule is possible only when there is an injury to the articular surface at the same time. This mechanism will be discussed in more detail later.

The mechanism which indirectly injures a meniscus is based almost always on a combination of sudden uncontrolled rotation and flexion-extension motions. This occurs either when the foot is fixed on the ground and the body makes a twisting motion, or the leg is rotated suddenly on a fixed femur. Although we know that minimal trauma in everyday living such as stumbling, skidding, tripping, or minor falls can tear a healthy, histologically intact meniscus, there are many specific activities which have a high incidence of meniscus lesions.

Most important of these are sports activities and first among these according to most authors is soccer followed by track and field and skiing. The following statistical analysis shows that there are considerable regional differences according to the popularity of the different sports.

It is evident that skiing is etiologically much more important in the alpine countries than in the flat countries. Percentagewise, however, soccer carries by far the highest incidence of meniscus lesions. Since the leg is usually well fixed to the lawn by the cleats on the soccer shoe, sudden changes of body position during passing, running, or collisions with fellow players can easily cause twisting motions in the knee joint (Fig. 11). In track and field the throwing and jumping events (hammer, discus, javelin, long jump, etc.) are particularly prone to meniscus lesions (Fig. 12a).

In skiing, also, the mechanism of injury is usually a twisting motion. This can occur when one ski suddenly slips or gets caught or when the body is abruptly turned (Fig. 12b). These

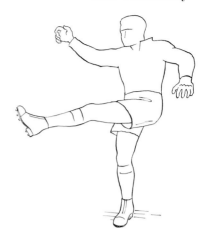

Fig. 11. Soccer player. Sudden torsion of the body against the fixed foot.

lesions are often combined with ligamentous damage, and the symptoms of ligamentous damage frequently predominate in fresh knee injuries from skiing. We have already mentioned that partial detachments and tears

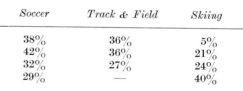

| Authors | | Soccer | Track & Field | Skiing |
|---|---|---|---|---|
| Groh | (Saarbrücken) | 38% | 36% | 5% |
| Bossard | (Swiss Accident Insurance Company) | 42% | 36% | 21% |
| Ritzmann | (Surgical University Clinic, Zurich) | 32% | 27% | 24% |
| Bestle | (Innsbruck) | 29% | — | 40% |

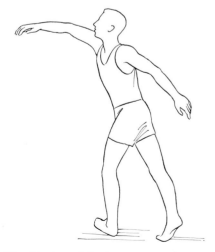

Fig. 12a. Torsion of the knee joint while throwing the discus.

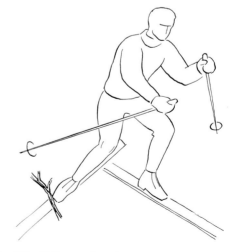

Fig. 12b. Skiing, a situation which can lead to tear of collateral ligament and/or meniscus lesion.

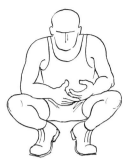

Fig. 13. Working in a squatting or kneeling position over a prolonged period of time can lead to pressure degeneration of the menisci.

of the menisci are not rare in skiing injuries. These lesions often do not heal, and minimal trauma not infrequently leads to typical locking after a long period of quiescence.

The percentage of *industrial injuries* in the total number of meniscus lesions also shows considerable regional variations. While Andreesen in his series of coal miners found 9 per cent sports injuries and 73 per cent industrial injuries, the ratio in Groh's series is exactly the reverse with 89 per cent sports injuries and 11 per cent industrial injuries. In the statistics of the Swiss Accident Insurance Company the number of meniscus lesions from industrial and non-industrial accidents is approximately the same (Bossard, Thurnherr). The mechanism of injury in industrial accidents is naturally more varied. Escape motions or attempts to protect against or avoid an external force predominate. Another known mechanism is the so-called swinging injury incurred especially while striking and missing with a heavy hammer (Groh).

Excessive wear of the menisci is found in activities where work is carried out in a kneeling or squatting position over a prolonged period of time. The continuous pressure causes pathologic degeneration of the menisci (Fig. 13). Foremost in this group are miners who have to work in low tunnels; however, floor layers, stone-cutters, gardeners, etc. are also affected.

Finally we should mention one other mechanism of injury which is frequently caused by *direct* violence and which seems to increase with the rising number of traffic accidents. These are *meniscus injuries associated* with *tibial plateau fractures*. We usually do not pay enough attention to the fact that every fracture of the tibia plateau with depression or step formation in the

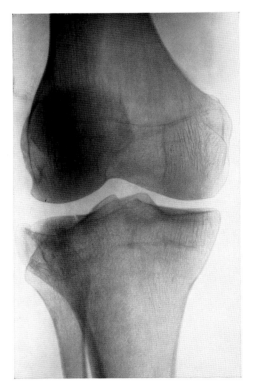

Fig. 14a. Fracture of the lateral tibial plateau with marked step formation and depression of the joint surface.

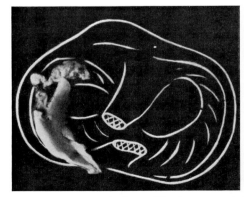

Fig. 14b. Operative findings. Massive tear of the lateral meniscus.

joint surface must automatically cause a detachment or tear of the meniscus. When these fractures are treated conservatively the concomitant meniscus injury is given little or no attention. Hoffmann and Stumpfegger, Schaer, and others have emphasized that overlooked meniscus lesions and adhesions of the meniscus at the fracture site are important reasons for residual disability and permanent impairment of function in conservatively treated tibial plateau fractures.

Most of the more severe fractures today are treated operatively and are reduced and fixed under vision. When we inspect the joint, we almost always find considerable damage to the meniscus. In our series of surgically treated tibial plateau fractures, which was published by Senn, we found concomitant injuries of one or both menisci in 70 per cent of the cases, while Andreesen, Hoffmann, and others report an incidence of 80 to 90 per cent. Since the lateral tibial plateau is fractured more frequently, the incidence of concomitant injuries to the lateral meniscus is also higher. Figure 14 shows a typical example. Whenever a fracture of the tibial plateau is treated surgically, the joint should always be inspected and the damaged meniscus removed. This approach will lead to a better functional result.

## 3) Typical Lesions

The findings which can be observed on the menisci during arthrotomy are manifold. The great majority consists of tears and ruptures, either perpendicular to the articular surface of the tibia or in an oblique direction. Small superficial tears are frequently located on the undersurface of the meniscus, as we have pointed out before.

Some of the typical tears which can occur in different variations and combinations are illustrated in figure 15.

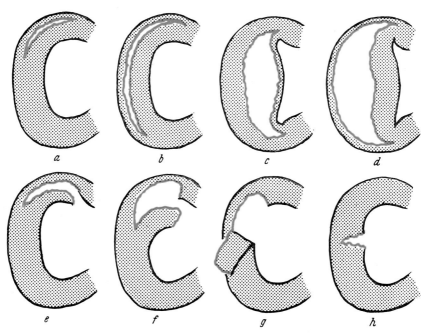

Fig. 15. Typical meniscus tears. a and b) Partial and subtotal longitudinal tear. c and d) Total longitudinal tear (bucket handle tear with displacement of the torn meniscus fragment into the interior of the joint). e and f) Tear of the anterior and posterior horn. g) Tongue-shaped tear with peripheral displacement. h) Transverse tear.

Most authors agree that the majority of meniscus lesions consist of *longitudinal tears* of the cartilaginous substance (one-half to two-thirds of all meniscus tears). When the tear reaches from the anterior or posterior horn beyond the attachment to the collateral ligament, the detached fragment can be displaced into the joint. This so-called *bucket-handle tear* is of considerable clinical significance because it is the only lesion which can cause true blockage or permanent locking of the knee joint. In most cases reposition of the displaced meniscus is possible by appropriate manipulation with or without anesthesia. In cases of recurrent locking, the patients usually learn to unlock their joint by certain motions such as forceful extension of the knee joint. Even if the displaced portion of the meniscus cannot be repositioned, normal motion usually returns after a certain period of time because the displaced bucket-handle eventually finds enough room in the intercondylar fossa.

The detached portion of the meniscus is frequently only a small sickle-shaped piece on the inner border. Occasionally, however, the entire meniscus can be detached from its attachment to the joint capsule and the collateral ligament. Most frequently the tear is located between the middle and outer third, and the well vascularized zone remains attached to the joint capsule.

Other typical lesions are detachments of the anterior or posterior horn or the simple transverse tears which occur more frequently in the lateral meniscus. In addition, there is a multiplicity of lobe- or-tongue shaped tears which can be caught between the condyles and cause temporary locking. Occasionally they are folded back towards the outside and can then be palpated between the joint capsule and the femoral condyle as a firm nodule which shifts with motion of the joint.

The significance of the so-called *hypermobile meniscus* is very controversial. It is frequently quite difficult to decide whether a certain relaxation of the attachments of the meniscus should be taken as a pathologic finding, or whether it is used as a convenient diagnosis because the clinically diagnosed meniscus lesion cannot be verified with arthrotomy. Smillie points out that stretching or tearing of the posterior meniscus attachment is the basis for the occurrence of a longitudinal tear. Most authors agree (Andreesen, Bircher, Schmidt, Groh, and others) that the hypermobile meniscus is a typical early form of the traumatic meniscus lesion and is produced by a tearing out or a gradual detachment of the meniscus from its attachments to capsule and ligaments. On the basis of many similar observations we agree with these authors that relaxation or detachment, especially of the posterior horn of the medial meniscus, is a characteristic finding which must be considered a precursor of the meniscus tear itself.

In contrast to traumatic lesions, degenerative changes of the menisci are usually classified under the heading *meniscopathy*. On the basis of the occasional histologic finding of small perivascular round cell infiltrations, Roux coined the term *"meniscitis."* We do not believe, however, that an inflammation of the meniscus as an independent pathologic picture exists. Inflammatory changes must be considered as changes coexisting with degenerative damage or generalized joint disease. We agree with Andreesen, Breitenfelder, Schaer, and others that meniscitis has nothing in common with the present concept of meniscus lesions and should be deleted from the nomenclature.

## 4) Classification of Meniscus Lesions

*"Meniscus lesion"* is a general term and does not allow conclusions as to the etiology of the damage. We know that a meniscus lesion can be caused by a multiplicity of factors such as trauma, ligamentous damage, degeneration, constitutional factors, etc. Evaluation for insurance companies have forced orthopedists and traumatologists to deal with these different factors and to classify lesions on an etiologic or pathologic basis. We do not attempt to add another classification to the many which are already in existence. The most useful classification in our opinion is that of Groh which was accepted by Buerkle de la Camp and Rostock for the *Handbuch für die gesamte Unfallheilkunde*. Groh's classification takes into consideration the history, the clinical and histologic findings, and also the temporal relationships.

According to Groh the following four groups can be distinguished:
1) Spontaneous detachment (meniscopathy, primary degeneration);
2) The fresh traumatic tear;
3) Late changes after traumatic tear (secondary degeneration);
4) Late changes after ligamentous damage (pseudo-primary degeneration).

The two most important etiological factors, trauma and degeneration, have been rated quite differently by different authors. Tobler was of the opinion that a normal healthy meniscus could not tear, but that degenerative changes would always precede the tear. Other authors consider trauma to be the most important etiologic factor (Burckhardt, Linde, and others). Present opinion gives consideration to both of these factors as can be seen in the classification of Groh.

Trauma unquestionably plays an important role in the etiology of meniscus lesions. During the period 1952–1953 the Swiss Accident Insurance Company accepted 485 out of 500 cases (97 per cent) as traumatic lesions (Bossard). Groh in his large series found spontaneous detachments in only 4 per cent of all cases. The much higher incidence of meniscus lesions among males and the fact that most meniscus lesions occur in the third and fourth decade also point to the etiologic importance of traumatic damage. If wear and tear and pathologic degeneration were important factors in the etiology of meniscus damage, we should find an increase in meniscus lesions in older age groups; this, however, is not the case.

Increased *wear and tear* does play a role in industrial and mining areas. Here we should consider pathologic degenerative changes as the primary cause (primary degeneration). The meniscus damage in these cases is caused primarily by the prolonged abnormal mechanical stress which is present in the so-called kneeling vocations.

Other factors, such as constitutional inferiority of the cartilaginous substance and generalized diseases of the knee joint (infections, arthritic changes), play only a small role in the etiology of meniscus lesions.

Primary degeneration leads to structural changes in the cartilaginous substance, and *predisposes to tears* (Henschen). A trivial, everyday motion such as straightening up from a squatting position or turning, even during sleep, can then lead to a *spontaneous tear* of the meniscus. These tears almost exclusively involve the medial meniscus. Single or multiple longitudinal tears, which almost always lie within the degenerated cartilaginous substance, are the rule. The knee joint reacts very little to this damage and usually shows only a moderate serous effusion.

A *fresh traumatic tear* with a characteristic injury usually presents a fairly clear-cut picture. A meniscus which is removed a few weeks after injury usually reveals bloody imbibitions. Histologic examination shows beginning repair with in-growing vessels and fibrocytes from the peripheral zone, but no significant degenerative changes.

Evaluation can be difficult when the meniscus lesion is caused by a trivial injury. The first injury to a "healthy meniscus" usually leads to a partial detachment from the joint capsule or a partial tear of the meniscus substance. Typical locking of the knee joint with dislocation of the meniscus into the joint is usually not seen with the first injury. The clinical symptoms are not very characteristic in the beginning and are frequently masked by concomitant ligamentous injuries. A peripheral meniscus injury close to the capsular attachment can heal with conservative treatment or quiet down sufficiently to make the patient free of symptoms during the subsequent weeks, months, or even years. An incompletely healed meniscus tear, on the other hand, can gradually enlarge with continued mechanical stress and lead to frequent locking of the knee even without additional injury. Use of the joint continuously traumatizes the torn part of the meniscus and causes degeneration of the tissue within a few weeks. These secondary degenerative changes are usually limited to the area of the tear but may be difficult to distinguish histologically from a tear through a degenerated meniscus. The same can be said for *late degenerative changes in an unstable knee.* The ligamentous instability of the joint causes continuous trauma to the meniscus and leads to progressive tissue degeneration and increased vulnerability. The degenerative process in these cases, however, is an indirect result of the usually traumatic ligamentous damage *(pseudo-primary* *degeneration)*. Degenerative changes in an unstable knee are not limited to the menisci, but also involve the joint cartilage and the joint capsule with chronic recurrent synovitis, infiltration of the infrapatellar fat pad, etc.

CHAPTER 3

# Clinical Diagnosis

There are a number of surgical conditions which sometimes can be diagnosed very easily. In other cases it may be very difficult to make a diagnosis and the diagnostic work-up may require a detailed history and a very thorough clinical examination. Internal derangement of the knee joint is one of these conditions. Occasionally the patient's description of his symptoms is sufficient to make a diagnosis of a bucket-handle tear of the medial meniscus. The majority of cases, however, present a complicated diagnostic problem which can be solved only by very thorough evaluation of all symptoms (Smillie). Schaer's statement that a diagnosis of meniscus lesion is never certain is still true today. Even experienced examiners often find that the operative diagnosis does not correspond with their clinical diagnosis.

One of the reasons for this diagnostic uncertainty is the fact that there are meniscus lesions which do not produce characteristic symptoms. This can be partially explained by the fact that the menisci do not have sensory nerve supply and symptoms are only produced when tears and irritations are present close to the joint capsule. Additionally, there are many posttraumatic conditions of the knee joint with symptoms difficult to distinguish from those of a damaged meniscus. We shall deal with the differential diagnosis of meniscus lesions in a separate paragraph.

In order to gain the necessary experience in the evaluation of knee joint symptoms, it is advisable to carry out the examination systematically with an established plan. The patient's history and clinical findings should always be written down. This permits a critical comparison of clinical and operative findings after surgery. Exact and good records are also of great importance for disability evaluation of a meniscus lesion.

## 1) History

We have already mentioned that it is sometimes possible to diagnose a meniscus lesion from the patient's history alone. An experienced traumatologist knows that a good history can tell as much, and occasionally more, about the nature of the patient's knee condition than the clinical examination. This makes a thorough and detailed history an absolute necessity for evaluation of an injured or diseased knee joint (Krömer).

The *time and the mechanism which produce the first symptoms* are very important factors. Quite often the symptoms can be related to a definite injury. Indirect injuries such as sudden uncontrolled rotary motions of the knee joint are characteristic for meniscus injuries. The mechanism of typical injuries has been discussed in previous chapters. The patient's own description of the injury, however, is frequently inaccurate and cannot be used for diagnosis. It is quite natural, for instance, for a patient to assume that hitting the knee on the ground produced the injury after he slipped on a wet surface and not the preceding sudden rotary motion of the knee joint. Thorough questioning of the patient will enlist his help in reconstructing the mechanism of the injury fairly accurately.

Sudden locking of the joint during an everyday activity such as climbing stairs, coming up from a squatting position, stumbling, or even turning over in bed without a definite injury should make us think of a spontaneous detachment of the meniscus or a late meniscus lesion from an old injury. The patient should always be questioned about his occupation because abnormal stress on the knee such as prolonged work in a kneeling position can produce degenerative changes in the meniscus. Quite frequently the patient will tell us that he had a knee injury a long time ago which was treated as a sprain and a meniscus lesion was not diagnosed.

## 2) Initial Symptoms

Almost all meniscus tears produce acute pain which is localized either in the joint space on the side of the injured meniscus or more diffusely in the whole knee joint. It may occasionally radiate into the lower leg. The nature of the pain will rarely permit us to distinguish a meniscus lesion from an injury to the capsular or ligamentous structures. A fresh, traumatic tear usually produces severe pain and immediate disability. The patient has to stop working and a soccer player is very rarely able to continue playing after suffering a tear of the meniscus. The patient with an acute sprain of the medial collateral ligament, on the other hand, will frequently be able to continue with some activity during the first few hours.

The rapidity with which *joint effusion* occurs after the knee injury can give us certain diagnostic clues. A massive and bloody effusion which forms within the first few hours after injury is usually produced by severe damage to the capsular or ligamentous structures or even the bones. Cartilaginous tissue is poorly vascularized and the effusion after a meniscus lesion develops slowly, sometimes not until the next day. Minor ligamentous injuries can also produce a serous effusion which develops slowly.

Spontaneous detachments of the menisci which occur without involvement of the joint capsule may not produce any effusion.

## 3) Locking

A history of locking is of great diagnostic significance. If the patient tells us that his knee locked in some degree of flexion after a minor injury and required forceful passive extension or even the help of other people to unlock it, we can make a diagnosis of meniscus tear from the history alone. The presence of loose bodies in the joint must be ruled out roentgenographically.

A torn meniscus produces locking of the joint when one fragment of the meniscus is caught between the condyles. The lesion frequently is a so-called bucket-handle tear with displacement of the bucket-handle into the joint. Displacement of a tongue-shaped fragment between the femoral condyle and the joint capsule can produce the same symptoms.

The blockage is never complete and the knee joint retains a limited range of motion against a rubbery resistance. Since occasionally limitation of motion from capsular contractures or joint effusions can produce the same symptoms, it is necessary to get an exact description of the locking mechanism. Frequently an audible "click" or "snap" is noticed. Classical locking produces limitation of extension of 20–45 degrees. When the knee is unlocked the patient usually has the impression that "something has slipped back to its normal place." With the exception of spontaneous detachment of an already damaged meniscus, classical locking is very rarely produced by the first injury. More often the patient tells us that originally he noticed only occasional minor snapping. These episodes became more frequent with time and eventually led to an episode of true locking. This description is indicative of a partial tear which gradually extended into a total longitudinal tear.

Sometimes the patient describes a sudden giving away of the leg instead of a true locking of the knee joint. This is a sudden disturbance "as if something snapped inside the joint." The "giving way" episodes are characteristic of momentary trapping of a meniscus fragment. They can also be true subluxations from cruciate or collateral ligament lesions, or from inadequate stability of the knee joint with insufficiency of the quadriceps. Detailed questioning of the patient and a thorough clinical examination will clarify the situation in most cases. We must mention, however, that not all meniscus lesions produce locking or "giving way" episodes. Our own series shows an incidence of locking in 82 per cent of all cases (Ritzmann). Smillie, on the other hand, found true locking in only 48 per cent of his cases. True locking, when present, however, is the most significant clinical symptom of a meniscus lesion.

### 4) Clinical Examination

When we are asked to evaluate a patient's knee symptoms, we should never limit our examination to the involved joint. Body build and general constitution, static and mechanics of the leg, development of the musculature, etc., are factors which must be taken into consideration. The involved extremity should always be compared with the normal opposite leg. Adolescents frequently project symptoms from pathology in the hip joint into the area of the knee. All these factors make an examination of both lower extremities of the disrobed patient mandatory. The condition of the thigh musculature is of special significance. Immobilization of the leg or favoring of the knee joint because of pain will produce a decrease in muscle volume and tone very rapidly, sometimes within one or two weeks. Atrophy of the quadriceps and especially of the vastus medialis is very rarely absent in a patient with a long-standing meniscus lesion. The vastus medialis is responsible for the last 10–15 degrees of extension. The painful limitation of extension which accompanies meniscus lesions frequently makes the vastus medialis ineffective and causes it to atrophy. Occasionally the remaining musculature of the thigh can undergo compensatory hypertrophy and mask atrophy of the vastus medialis when we measure

the circumference of the thigh. Inspection or palpation of the contracted quadriceps during straight leg raising or standing will make atrophy of the vastus medialis apparent in these cases.

Inspection will reveal abnormal swelling, changes of contour, skin color or scars from previous injuries or operations. Palpation will help us clarify the nature of a joint swelling. Comparison of both knee joints will reveal an increase in skin temperature from an irritation of the joint. Posttraumatic extra-articular soft tissue swellings and hematomata point to injuries of the capsule and/or the collateral ligaments. Diffuse infiltration of the joint capsule is always due to a long-standing irritation or inflammatory process and is one of the late changes after a meniscus lesion.

A *joint effusion* can be best shown by "ballottement of the patella." The joint is placed in full extension and the patient is asked to relax his muscles. The examining finger can then press the patella down on the femoral condyles. Upon release of pressure it will immediately return to its original position. When the effusion is small, ballottement of the patella can be produced by placing the knee on a pillow and compressing the suprapatellar pouch (Fig. 16). Meniscus lesions frequently produce effusion of the joint. Neither the presence of a joint effusion nor its composition permit definite diagnostic conclusions. A bloody effusion after an injury to the knee joint only means that blood vessels have been injured. This can occur with injury to the vascularized portion of the meniscus or any other vascularized internal structures

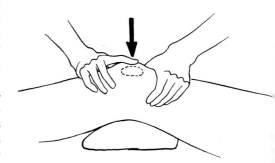

Fig. 16. Demonstration of *knee joint effusion*. Pressure over the suprapatellar pouch will permit ballottement of the patella even with small effusions.

of the knee joint. Small fat droplets in the effusion indicate a concomitant bony injury.

The old dictum that every meniscus injury produces a bloody joint effusion is no longer valid. A tear in the non-vascularized inner zone of the meniscus can only produce a serous effusion. Minor meniscus lesions, extension of an old partial tear, or spontaneous detachment of the meniscus can occur without any effusion. Limitation of extension against a rubbery resistance is considered a classical symptom of a meniscus lesion. In most cases this is due to entrapment of the torn meniscus fragment. Incomplete tears or crushing of the meniscus can also lead to reflex limitation of extension because the damaged meniscus is placed under tension or pressure when the knee is extended. Painful limitation of extension is not characteristic of a meniscus lesion. Chronic irritation of the knee joint always leads to a certain limitation of extension due to increased tension and infiltration of the joint capsule. The same is true of fresh injuries to the collateral and cruciate ligaments because full extension tightens the ligaments and produces pain. Damage to the meniscus usually does not impair flexion of the knee joint in contrast to injuries of the capsular and ligamentous structures. Examination of the liga-

ments is mandatory. We have already mentioned that a meniscus lesion is frequently accompanied by a ligamentous injury, especially of the medial collateral and the anterior cruciate ligaments. Proper evaluation of the collateral ligaments is possible only with the knee in full extension. Mild lateral instability in the presence of an extension lack can be within normal limits, especially when there is marked atrophy of the quadriceps.

Relaxation of the cruciate ligaments can be demonstrated with the so-called *drawer sign* (Fig. 17). The patient is asked to relax his musculature and flex his knee to a right angle. The examiner then grasps the lower leg with both hands and pushes it forward and backward in the sagittal plane. Displacement of the tibia anteriorly of more than 4 to 5 mm. is indicative of a lesion of the anterior cruciate ligament. Abnormal posterior displacement of the tibia which would indicate a rupture of the posterior cruciate ligament is rare.

Constant localized *tenderness* can be a valuable diagnostic sign. A lesion of the medial meniscus quite often produces tenderness in the anterior half of the medial joint line, one to two fingerbreadths anterior to the medial collateral ligament. A similar tenderness localized in the lateral joint line indicates a lesion of the lateral meniscus. Tenderness in the posterior portion of the joint line is found less frequently.

We know from experience that the point of greatest tenderness is not necessarily identical with the location of the meniscus lesion. Tenderness in the anteromedial joint line can be present with ruptures of the middle portion, the posterior horn or with a complete longitudinal tear of medial meniscus and occasionally with a lesion of the lateral meniscus. We have no explanation for this latter finding which can make diagnosis of the meniscus lesion extremely difficult.

Occasionally palpation of the joint line reveals increased resistance or a tender ridge which represents the damaged swollen meniscus (Nicolet). This finding should not be confused with a partial tear of the anterior horn with the fragment dislocated to the outside. This protrusion can usually be palpated only with the joint in

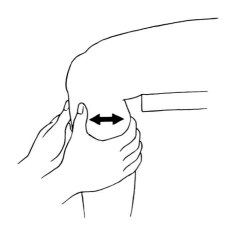

Fig. 17. Demonstration of the *"drawer sign."* Anterior displacement of the tibia in relation to the fixed thigh of more than 5 mm. indicates lesion of the anterior cruciate ligament. Similar posterior displacement indicates lesion of the posterior cruciate ligament which is much rarer.

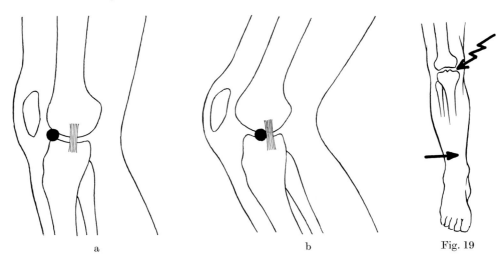

a                                                    b                           Fig. 19

Fig. 18. *Second Steinmann's sign:* Flexion of the knee joint displaces a point of tenderness over the anterior joint line towards the collateral ligament.

Fig. 19. *Böhler's sign:* Pain in the medial joint space on abduction of the tibia indicates lesion of the medial meniscus. Pain in the lateral joint space on abduction of the tibia indicates lesion of the lateral meniscus.

complete extension and disappears with flexion of the knee. A rubbery cystic bulge which does not move usually represents a ganglion of the meniscus. These are more frequent on the lateral side of the knee joint.

## 5) Meniscus Signs

A great number of special diagnostic signs have been described for the diagnosis of meniscus lesions. Most of these tests are known by the author's name and can be very helpful in differentiating meniscus lesions from other lesions of the knee joint. All of these so-called meniscus signs can help us diagnose a meniscus lesion when they are positive. A negative maneuver, however, does not necessarily mean that the meniscus is intact. Most of these tests are so similar that it is immaterial which maneuver is used. It is important, however, that the examiner always use the same tests because the accuracy of diagnosis improves with increasing experience. Following is a list of several of the better known meniscus signs. This list is by no means complete.

### a) 2nd Steinmann's Sign

This sign was described by Steinmann of Bern and can usually be carried out without much difficulty. It is useful in all cases where localized tenderness is present in the anterior joint line. Flexion of the knee joint will displace the point of tenderness in the direction of the collateral ligament; extension will displace it anteriorly when a meniscus lesion is present. Knee flexion displaces the menisci posteriorly on the tibial plateau and tenderness which arises from a meniscus lesion will move in the same direction. A painful arthrotic spur on the tibial plateau, on the other hand, would not change its position with flexion and extension.

### b) Bragard's Sign

This test also depends on the presence of a point of tenderness in the anterior joint line. Internal rotation and extension of the tibia will increase the tenderness from a lesion of the medial meniscus because this motion pushes the meniscus against the examining finger. Frequently a palpable increase in resistance can be noted. External rotation and flexion of the tibia

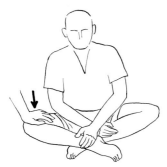

Fig. 20. *Payr's sign:* The so-called "turkish seat" produces pain when a lesion of the posterior horn of the medial meniscus is present.

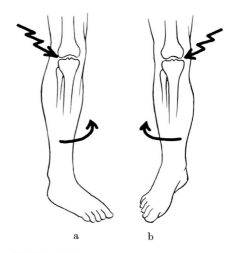

a                    b

Fig. 21. *First Steinmann's sign:* Pain in the lateral joint space with *internal rotation* of the flexed tibia indicates lesion of the *lateral* meniscus (a). Pain in the medial joint space with *external* rotation of the flexed tibia indicates lesion of the *medial* meniscus (b).

on the other hand, displace the meniscus into the joint, and pressure from the examiner's finger causes less or no pain. A similar test can be used for lesions of the lateral meniscus.

### c) Böhler's Sign

Böhler has shown that narrowing of the medial joint space (adduction) will cause pain when a lesion of the medial meniscus is present whereas narrowing of the lateral joint space (abduction) is painful with a lesion of the lateral meniscus (Fig. 19). Experience has shown that this sign is not very reliable. Krömer recommends that the knee be flexed and extended in forced adduction or abduction. This increases the possibility of compressing the injured part of the meniscus. It can occasionally produce locking when a tongue-shaped tear is present. Krömer has described another modification of the test. He recommends flexion and extension of the knee in both forced adduction and abduction. With a lesion of the medial meniscus, adduction should cause pain and locking; abduction should decompress the meniscus and cause the symptoms to decrease or disappear.

### d) Payr's Sign

This test produces pressure on the middle and posterior portions of the medial meniscus. The patient is asked to assume a so-called turkish sitting position. The examiner then applies pressure on the knee joint (Fig. 20). Pain on the medial side of the knee joint is indicative of a

lesion of the posterior horn of the medial meniscus.

### e) 1st Steinmann's Sign

The knee is flexed to a right angle and the tibia forcefully rotated externally and internally. Pain in the medial joint space on external rotation is indicative of a lesion of the medial meniscus, whereas pain in the lateral joint space on internal rotation indicates a lesion of the lateral meniscus. This sudden rotation causes displacement of the meniscus into the joint and produces a painful pull on the torn meniscus. We recommend repeating the test several times in different positions of flexion.

### f) Merke's Sign

This sign is similar to the 1st Steinmann's sign, but rotations are carried out with the patient standing. The patient is asked to rotate his body on the fixed leg internally and externally. This compresses the menisci and the pain on rotation is usually more intense than with Steinmann's test. Pain in the medial joint space on internal rotation of the body indicates a lesion of the medial meniscus.

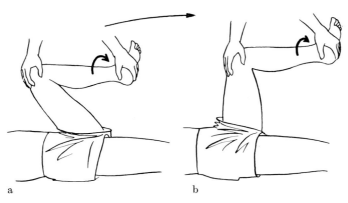

a                                      b

Fig. 22. *McMurray test* (Fig. 22a): For evaluation of the medial meniscus: Phase 1. Hip and knee joint of the involved leg are markedly flexed and the foot *externally* rotated. Phase 2. (Fig. 22b): The externally rotated leg is gradually extended beyond a right angle.
Evaluation of the *lateral* meniscus is carried out in a similar manner with the leg in internal rotation.

### g) McMurray Test

This test is very popular in the Anglo-Saxon countries and permits detection of tears in the middle and posterior parts of the menisci fairly accurately. With the patient in a supine position, hip and knee joints are flexed markedly until the heel almost touches the buttock. The examiner holds and fixes the knee joint with one hand and manipulates the foot with the other hand. For evaluation of the medial meniscus the foot is rotated externally and the knee joint then extended while external rotation of the tibia is maintained (Fig. 22). Examination of the lateral meniscus is carried out with the tibia in internal rotation. If this maneuver produces an audible or palpable snap in the joint, a tear of the meniscus is usually present. This extreme flexion and rotation displaces the meniscus into the joint and limits its mobility to a point where it has to move with the tibia. Extension of the tibia then moves the torn fragment of the meniscus over the femoral condyle and produces a snap. The test frequently permits localization of the lesion with good accuracy. A tear in the posterior horn produces a snap in marked flexion, a tear in the middle portion produces a snap at approximately 90 degrees. One advantage of this test is that it is not dependent on producing pain because older tears in the substance of the meniscus frequently do not cause pain.

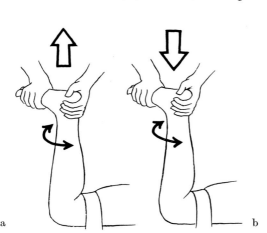

a                                      b

Fig. 23. *Apley test:* a) Distraction test: Pain in the knee on rotation of the foot under traction indicates damage to the capsule and the ligamentous structures. b) Compression test: Pain and snapping in the knee on rotation of the foot under pressure indicate lesion of the meniscus.

### h) Apley Test

This test is not widely known on the continent. Its main advantage is a differentiation of meniscus lesions from lesions of the capsule and ligaments. With the patient in a prone position, the knee is flexed 90 degrees and the tibia then rotated internally and externally with manual traction on the foot (Fig. 23a). Pain with this test usually indicates a lesion of the capsule and ligaments. The test is then repeated but pressure is applied to the foot and thus to the joint surfaces of the knee (Fig. 23b). Pain and snapping with this test usually indicate a lesion of the medial meniscus as with the McMurray test. By doing this maneuver in different positions of flexion, the different sections of the meniscus can be examined separately.

In addition to the special meniscus tests, the

knee should be examined for degenerative changes in the articular surfaces (arthrosis), the patella (chondromalacia), the infrapatellar fat pad (Hoffa's disease), and changes in the popliteal fossa (bursae and cysts). Crepitus and other audible signs can be of diagnostic significance. We will discuss these changes in more detail in the section on differential diagnosis.

Mention must be made here of one other phenomenon, the so-called *snapping knee*. This is an audible snap inside the knee joint which is produced regularly with flexion or extension. This phenomenon is usually observed in adolescents and may be due to developmental anomalies (ring or discoid meniscus), cystic degeneration or a traumatic lesion of the lateral meniscus. Occasionally it is due to a tendon which snaps over a bony prominence in the tibia or over the head of the fibula.

In the majority of cases we will be able to diagnose a meniscus lesion with accuracy on the basis of the patient's history and a thorough clinical examination. If we are unable to clarify the diagnosis, however, we should make it a rule to supplement our clinical evaluation by X-ray examination and arthrography.

CHAPTER 4

# Routine X-Ray Examination of the Knee

Roentgen examination with routine anterior/posterior and lateral views is indicated for all posttraumatic knee lesions. X-rays should be taken not only when the symptoms are not clear but also when a meniscus lesion is suspected or even when the meniscus lesion is obvious. The X-ray can give us information about changes in bone and cartilage such as fractures, inflammation, tumors, bony anomalies, and degenerative lesions such as chondromalacia, chondromatosis, or osteochondritis.

Soft tissue lesions of the knee can sometimes be evaluated in their late stages with conventional X-ray views (e.g., Pellegrini-Stieda's lesion). (See Fig. 177.) Avulsions of the tibial spines will help in the evaluation of cruciate ligament lesions. Calcifications in the infrapatellar and the dorsal fat pad as well as the bursae can be visualized (see Fig. 198). Villous synovitis can lead to cystic lesions in the bone, especially in the area of the intercondylar fossa (Bessler-Rüttimann). (See Fig. 201.) Even relatively small intra-articular effusions from a synovitis or posttraumatic hemarthrosis can be visualized on the lateral view as soft tissue shadows, especially in the suprapatellar pouch. They can also produce a ventral displacement of the more radiolucent infrapatellar fat pad. Small intra-articular fractures can occasionally be visualized by Holmgren's method, which is a lateral view of the knee joint with the patient in the supine position and the X-ray beam directed horizontally. The fracture causes extrusion of blood and bone marrow fat into the knee joint. The lighter, more radiolucent fat floats on top of the blood and the borderline between the two can be visualized (Fig. 24).

Routine X-ray examination is of limited diagnostic value in the evaluation of meniscus lesions. It can help us visualize calcification of the meniscus (Fig. 25), erosions of bone from a meniscus ganglion (Jonasch; see Fig. 204), and secondary arthrotic changes from primary meniscus lesions (see Figs. 185, 186). Rauber and Lindbloom have described a sign which should be mentioned here. It consists of a bony spur on the tibial plateau adjacent to the damaged meniscus which is localized to the area of the meniscus lesion. The remaining sections of the joint do not show any arthrotic changes.

Traction on the joint can produce intra-articular gas. This method was utilized by Dittmar,

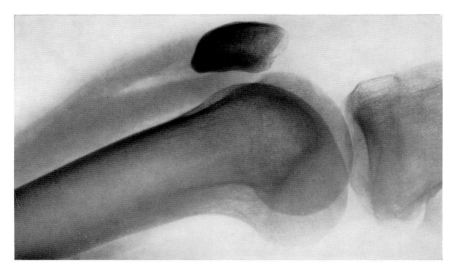

Fig. 24. Lateral view of the knee joint. Depressed fracture of the lateral tibial plateau. *Holmgren*'s *sign:* Layer formation in the suprapatellar pouch: Free bone marrow fat floats on top of the blood.

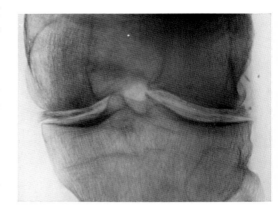

Magnusson and Long for a kind of gas arthrography. It can be helpful in detecting large meniscus lesions but is of no value for a detailed examination.

Fig. 25. Calcification of the medial and lateral meniscus.

CHAPTER 5

# Arthrography

## A. Historical Review

Wernerdorff and Robinson showed the first air arthrograms of the knee joint at the fourth German Orthopedic meeting in 1905, just 10 years after discovery of the roentgen rays. One year later Hoffa and Rauenbusch published their first experiences with arthrograms following injection of pure oxygen into the knee joint.

No significant contributions were made during the following decades. It was not until 1930 and later that the two Swiss surgeons, Bircher and Oberholzer, published their pioneer work with double contrast arthrography. Krömer, Laarmann and Boehm also made contributions in this field. Other authors such as Guerin, Ulrich, Giacobbe, Terracol and Colaneri, Chauvin, Anzillotti, Schum, Junghagen, Simon, Hamilton and Farrington, Stark, Judet, Archimbaud, Merle D'Aubigné, Serra de Oliveira, Möhlmann and Madlener, Meschan and McGave worked with air and oxygen arthrography. Arthrography with a liquid contrast medium was popularized by such authors as Colp and Klingenstein, Michaelis, Stocker, Stör, Boyd, Schüller, Nagy and Polgar, Lagergreen, Canigiani and Pirker, Palmer, Buss and Schaer, and Fischer. We must also mention the excellent papers by Lindblom and Ficat. Further contributions in the field of double contrast arthrography were made by Van de Berg and Crevecoeur, Croonenbergh and Rombouts, Candardjis, Rüttimann, Del Buono, Catolla, and Cavalcanti.

## B. Introduction and Indications

We have used the double contrast method exclusively for arthrography of the knee joint for several years now. We prefer this method to air arthrography which we have used earlier, and to arthrography with a liquid contrast medium alone. The technic is relatively easy to use, and we find that the method gives the best details and is not difficult to evaluate for both radiologist and surgeon. In our experience arthrography of the knee joint is indicated in the following conditions:

1) To evaluate all unclear knee symptoms with or without trauma, especially when there is considerable discrepancy between the subjective complaints and the objective findings.

2) When there is difficulty in localizing the meniscus lesion either to the medial or lateral meniscus.

3) In fresh ligamentous tears when an additional meniscus lesion cannot be ruled out.

4) Status after meniscectomy with persistent symptoms.

5) Documentation in disability evaluation.

## C. Methodology

### 1) Materials

The following materials are used for double contrast arthrography as shown in Fig. 26:

1) A razor;

2) Several sponges;

3) A sponge clamp;

4) Ether to defat the skin;

5) A skin disinfectant;

6) Local anesthetic;

7) A 5 cc. syringe and a 25 gauge needle for local anesthesia;

8) A 20 cc. syringe and 2 large caliber needles, 2″ long, for joint aspiration and injection of the contrast media (air and liquid contrast medium);

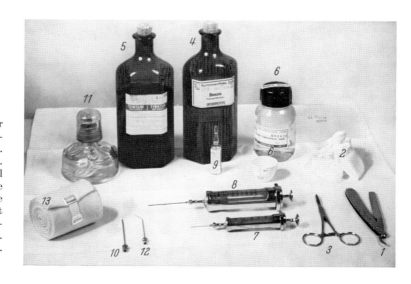

Fig. 26. Instruments for double contrast arthrography. 1. Razor. 2. Sponges. 3. Sponge clamp. 4. Ether. 5. Skin disinfectant. 6. Local anesthetic. 7. 5-cc. syringe with needle. 8. 20-cc. syringe with needle. 9. Contrast medium. 10. Aspiration needle. 11. Alcohol burner. 12. Second injection needle. 13. Elastic bandage.

9) Liquid contrast medium (4 to 5 cc. ampule);

10) Large caliber needle to aspirate the liquid contrast medium;

11) Alcohol burner to singe off the edge of the ampule before aspiration of the liquid contrast medium;

12) A second needle to remove the air at the end of the examination;

13) An elastic bandage.

## 2) Contrast Media

For double contrast arthrography we use two contrast media, air and a liquid *water-soluble contrast medium*. In the beginning pure oxygen was used for gas arthrography but it was soon found that normal atmospheric air was tolerated without complications. The air can be aspirated into the syringe over an alcohol flame. We use this manipulation very rarely and have never seen a complication from contaminated air.

We have tried most of the commercially available water-soluble contrast media. For many years we used the 50 per cent di-iodide Joduron which gave a relatively good contrast and was tolerated well. A tri-iodide dye will give even more intensive and better contrast. The dye must not be too viscous; otherwise the film will become too thick and obscure finer details. We have found the tri-iodide Opacoron (Cilag, Schaffhausen) to be very useful. It provides excellent contrast and is tolerated well. We usually inject 3 to 5 cc. of contrast medium according to the size of the joint. Larger amounts of contrast medium produce disturbing dye collections and the formation of air bubbles. Excess contrast medium frequently fills the bursae connected with the joint and creates a disturbing superimposition of contrast medium.

## 3) Technic

Exact and standardized technic is a prerequisite for good results with arthrography.

### a) Puncture of the Joint

Patients with stiff muscles and inelastic joints should loosen up with a few exercises, either

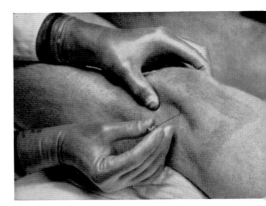

Fig. 27. Insertion of needle from the lateral side. The needle is inserted into the joint while the examiner's other hand pushes the patella to the lateral side to widen the patellar-femoral joint space.

actively or passively, before the joint is punctured. This will facilitate the entire examination.

The knee is first shaved, then defatted with ether and is cleansed with a disinfectant three times. The joint is punctured under local anesthesia of skin and joint capsule. A needle approximately two inches long and not too thick (approximately one millimeter in diameter) with a short bevel is used. If we use heavier needles air can escape through the puncture wound into the surrounding soft tissues after removal of the needle. The joint is punctured from the lateral side (Fig. 27). The examiner's hand moves the patella laterally to widen the joint space between patella and femoral condyle. The needle is then inserted between the articular surfaces of the patella and the femur until the needle hits the articular cartilage of the patella. The needle is then withdrawn slightly (approximately 1 mm.) and its tip is now located within the joint cavity. Joint fluid can be aspirated and air can be injected and withdrawn without resistance. Anesthesia of the joint itself is not necessary. When painful locking of the joint is present the injection of some anesthetic solution into the joint can be useful. An occasional patient with marked pain in the medial joint space on motion and especially extension will benefit from additional local anesthesia of the painful area.

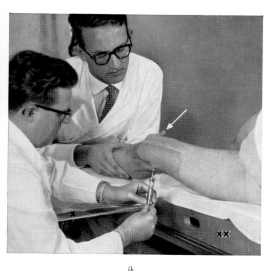

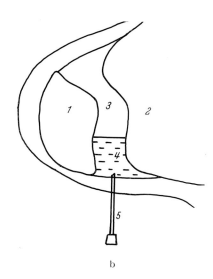

a                                               b

Fig. 28. Aspiration of a knee joint effusion in left lateral position. a) The patient is positioned on the X-ray table on a wooden frame (xx). The foot is placed on a small table (x). The needle is inserted in a vertical direction. The posterior joint space is compressed by an assistant (arrow). b) Schematic drawing of the patellar-femoral space during aspiration. 1. Patella. 2. Femoral condyle. 3. Air injected into the upper patellar femoral joint space. 4. Joint fluid in the patellar femoral joint space. 5. The tip of the needle is just inside the joint space.

## b) Evacuation of Joint Effusion

If a joint effusion is present it must be aspirated before the contrast media are injected, even when only a few cubic centimeters are present. Aspiration of the joint fluid with the patient in supine position is often difficult and one cannot be sure that all excess joint fluid has been evacuated. Complete evacuation of joint effusions is necessary for good quality of the arthrogram to avoid dilution of the contrast medium. We use a simple and rapid method to aspirate the joint with the patient in the lateral position (Fig. 28). First we inject approximately 10 cc. of air into the joint; the patient is then positioned on the affected side and places the foot of the affected leg on a small table adjacent to the examining table. Pressure is applied on the popliteal space and the joint fluid can now be aspirated without difficulty. Toward the end of the aspiration the needle may have to be withdrawn until its tip is just protruding through the synovial membrane. This places the tip of the needle into the lowest point of the fluid collection and makes it possible to aspirate even large effusions within a short period of time.

## c) Injection of Contrast Media

We first inject air into the joint followed by injection of the liquid contrast medium. Injection of the air should meet no resistance if the needle is correctly placed. In case of poor placement of the needle, air injected into the periarticular tissues will disturb evaluation of the arthrogram less than contrast medium injected into the periarticular tissues.

We first inject approximately 40 cc. of air with a 20 cc. syringe. A three-way valve or an elastic tube which can be clamped between syringe and needle are usually not necessary. Even though we may lose a little air when we change syringes, the joint will still be distended adequately. There should be no pain from excessive distention. We then inject approximately 3 to 4 cc. of liquid contrast medium and withdraw the needle. Rubbing the point of injection with a sterile sponge will compress the puncture wound and prevent the air from escaping. The patient is then allowed to sit up and the examiner moves the knee joint passively in extension, flexion, and rotation. We also let the patient stand up on the healthy leg to assure good coverage of the distal parts of the joint with contrast medium. All internal structures of the knee joint are now evenly covered with a thin film of liquid contrast medium. Small collections of contrast medium occasionally form in the posterior joint space. This, however, does not interfere with evaluation of the arthrogram. When ligamentous and capsular tears are present the contrast medium can escape into the soft tissues which will permit the diagnosis of these lesions (see page 95).

The air is usually removed from the joint at the end of the examination. The patient is advised to rest the leg for approximately half a day or a full day and should bandage the knee with an Ace bandage for several days. Disturbing noises which are occasionally present will disappear after a few days.

### 4) Equipment

The X-ray tube should have a very small focal spot (0.3 mm.²) to insure maximum detail in the visualization of the meniscus. If this tube is not available, we recommend insertion of a fine grain grid into the casette similar to those used for bone X-ray examination.

We have attached a wooden frame of approximately 15 cm. height to the fluoroscopy table. The patient lies on this frame. The thigh of the affected leg is supported by two to three pillows to facilitate rotation of the leg around its longitudinal axis during examination (see Fig. 30). The use of this wooden frame and the pillows increases the focus to object distance by 20 cm. from 70 to 90 cm. This improves the quality of the X-ray picture considerably and facilitates examination of the bony structures.

### 5) Physical Basis for Meniscus Visualization

The meniscus is best visualized when its longitudinal axis lies tangentially to the direction of the rays (see Fig. 29). Its projection on the fluoroscopy screen is then orthograde and

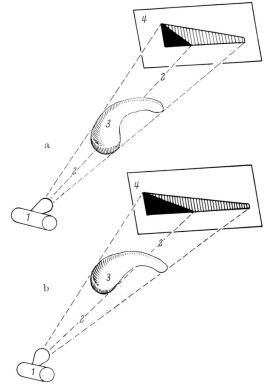

Fig. 29. Principles of meniscus visualization during arthrography. 1. X-ray tube 2. Central ray 3. Meniscus with one zone tangentially or orthograde to the central ray. 4. X-ray cassette or fluoroscopy screen a) the cross section of the orthograde portion of the middle zone of the meniscus is black. The image of the remaining portions of the meniscus is crosshatched. b) The meniscus is rotated to visualize the posterior horn in an orthograde position.

visualization on the film is clear. X-ray projection of the meniscus is in the shape of a wedge with the wedge representing the cross section of the meniscus at the point where it is tangential or orthograde to the central ray. When the central ray is directed tangentially to the middle zone of the meniscus as in figure 29 a, the projection of this middle zone will be sharp on the fluoroscopy screen. The other portions of the meniscus can also be visualized but are blurry. If the central ray is directed tangentially at the posterior horn, projection of the posterior horn will be sharp; the remaining portions of the meniscus will be blurry or not visualized at all

(Fig. 29 b). This explains why lesions of the meniscus that are tangential to the direction of the ray, such as longitudinal tears, are visualized clearly whereas transverse tears are usually blurry.

## 6) X-ray Technic

The patient is positioned under fluoroscopy for all views to insure orthograde projection of the meniscus on the film. The fluoroscopy unit is in a horizontal position. The patient lies first in a prone position on the wooden frame mentioned above (see Fig. 30). The examiner now rotates the patient's leg around its longitudinal axis under fluoroscopy while a technician shoots the X-ray views in the desired position. Since both menisci cannot be projected orthograde at the same time, each meniscus must be fluoroscoped separately. The planes of both menisci are not congruent because the medial and lateral tibial plateaus form an angle which can vary considerably.

### a) Visualization of the Medial Meniscus

Slight abduction of the tibia will open the medial joint space and allow free projection of the medial meniscus (Fig. 30). The meniscus can be seen on the fluoroscopy screen as a sharply outlined wedge. Care must be taken to obtain good delineation of the tibial surface of the meniscus from the articular surface of the tibia. With proper positioning the space between the meniscus and the tibia is seen as an air-containing strip on the fluoroscopy screen which will insure orthograde projection of the meniscus. Exact positioning of the meniscus is only possible with fluoroscopy. After optimal projection of the different meniscus sections has been obtained, X-ray exposures are then made in the desired positions. These positions are distributed over the entire length of the meniscus, which is examined stepwise in a ventral to dorsal direction.

Visualization of the anterior horn of the medial meniscus is easier with the knee in slight

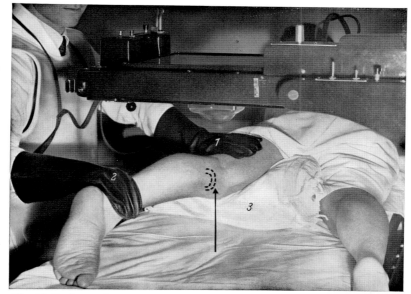

Fig. 30. Position of the patient and X-ray technic for visualization of the media meniscus. The patient is in the prone position. The examiner observes through the fluoroscopy screen and rotates the leg with his hands into the desired positions. Both hands are protected with lead gloves. The left hand (1) holds the thigh, the right hand (2) abducts the leg. The interrupted lines represent the medial meniscus. The vertical arrow corresponds to the central ray. 3. Pillow.

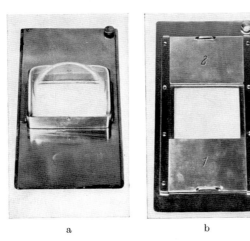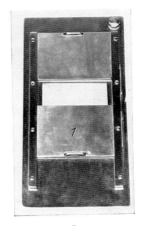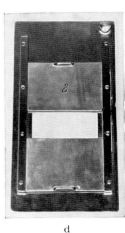

a                    b                    c                    d

Fig. 31. a) Regular spot film cassette. b) Modified spot film cassette; the plastic cover has been removed. Lower (1) and upper sliding cover (2). c) Position of sliding covers for the first series; upper half of the cassette exposed. d) Position of sliding covers for the second series on the same film; lower half of cassette exposed.

flexion, whereas the posterior horn is best seen with the knee in complete extension. A flexion contracture can occasionally lead to poor projection of the posterior horn. However, these patients do not usually require arthrography because incomplete extension of the knee after trauma is usually an indication for surgery. Occasionally arthrography is indicated in these cases either to localize a loose body or to determine whether the medial or the lateral meniscus is injured. Usually the limitation of extension is not very painful and the knee joint can be extended passively far enough to make visualization of the posterior horn possible.

### b) Visualization of the Lateral Meniscus

This is done in the same manner as that of the medial meniscus. The lateral joint space can usually be opened without difficulty by adduction of the tibia. Occasionally slight rotation or flexion of the tibia in addition to abduction or adduction is indicated for optimal orthograde projection of the menisci. The space between meniscus and tibia will show up even better in this position. Sometimes slight rotation may be added for better visualization of certain lesions. With increasing experience the examiner will be able to visualize the space between meniscus and tibia without any difficulty and can then project the meniscus orthograde in its entire circumference very rapidly so that the entire arthrogram can be done in a few minutes.

### c) Multiple Views

Using the spot film cassette and fluoroscopy four to six spot views can be taken depending on the cassette. We have modified our four-spot film cassette in such a way to enable us to take eight exposures on the same film, which reduces the amount of film material used in arthrography by about half (see Fig. 31). The aperture of our spot film cassette which was 10.5 cm. wide and 9.5 cm. long was reduced by two sliding covers to one-half of the length. The lower cover will cover the lower half of the aperture and the upper covers the upper half. Accordingly, only the open field will be visualized on the fluoroscopy screen or the film (see Figs. 31 b, c, d). This method enables us to produce eight exposures of 4.75 cm. by 10.5 cm. on one film.

We can thus visualize the affected meniscus in eight to ten different positions in its entire circumference (see Fig. 32). The entire length of the meniscus is approximately 5 cm. which is examined by 10 different views. This will give us 10 cross sections of the meniscus 5 mm. apart and enables us to show even small lesions. We recommend multiple spot film exposures for the more frequently injured posterior horn of the medial meniscus and the anterior horn of the lateral meniscus. With increasing experience the examiner will be able to detect larger meniscus lesions under fluoroscopy. We consider this relatively high number of exposures to be absolutely necessary. As a rule we take fewer exposures of the lateral meniscus then of the medial unless the lateral meniscus is suspect of injury.

### d) Visualization of Other Intra-articular Structures

Multiple views of the menisci should be supplemented by a lateral view of the entire joint in slight flexion. A lateral X-ray of the knee in flexion of approximately 30 to 45 degrees with minimal internal rotation gives an excellent view of the cruciate ligaments (Fig. 33). These views can be made with the regular X-ray tube which produces more detailed pictures. Good visualization of the cruciate ligaments can also be obtained with the knee at approximately 45 degrees of flexion and the patient in the supine position with a curved film cassette placed into the popliteal space (Fig. 34). On the lateral view we can also visualize the other joint spaces such as the suprapatellar pouch, the infrapatellar fat pad, the posterior fat pad and occasionally also the bursae. Axial views of the patella can be added if necessary (Fig. 35). The articular surface of the patella can be seen well on the lateral view, but occasionally may show up better with the knee in full extension (Fig. 36). *Tomograms* have not been used very much for examination of the menisci but can be very valuable for examination of the articular surface of the patella (Fuermaier) and for localization of loose bodies.

### 7) Technical Errors

*Periarticular* injection of the liquid contrast medium occurs most frequently into the loose fatty tissue between the anterior surface of the femur and the posterior wall of the suprapatellar pouch (superior recessus). The result is a dense, irregular shadow of contrast medium (Fig. 37). This makes a second injection of liquid contrast medium with subsequent passive motion necessary.

Periarticular or excessive injection of air leads to emphysema of the soft tissues (Fig. 38). The serosal cover of the inner surface of the knee joint is rather delicate and can easily be torn by excessive pressure in the joint, resulting in extrusion of air into the soft tissues. The use of an open needle reduces the risk of excessive pressure considerably and the joint capsule will not be extended to a point where it causes pain, for which the patient is usually grateful. Excessive air can always escape through the open needle before the last 20 cc. are injected.

## D. The Normal Arthrogram

### 1) The Normal Meniscus

The normal meniscus presents itself in an orthograde projection as a homogeneous wedge-shaped shadow of soft tissue density whose pointed edge is directed toward the interior of the joint. The angle of the inner corner is always acute, never obtuse. The tibial and femoral surfaces of the meniscus are always smooth and due to the thin film of dye which covers them present as thin sharply delineated borders (Fig. 39). These contours are normally slightly concave with the concavity usually greater on the femoral than on the tibial surface (Fig. 40). If the concavity on the femoral surface of the meniscus is more marked, degenerative changes should be suspected (see page 71). Convex contours of the meniscus are rare (see Fig. 43).

The base of the meniscal wedge usually blends into the capsular shadow without interruption. Occasionally so-called recessus are found in these areas. They can occur on the femoral or on the tibial surface or on both at the same time (Figs. 41 and 42). The size of these recessus varies but they are usually short and localized to the posterior horn on the medial side or to the anterior horn on the lateral side. We have

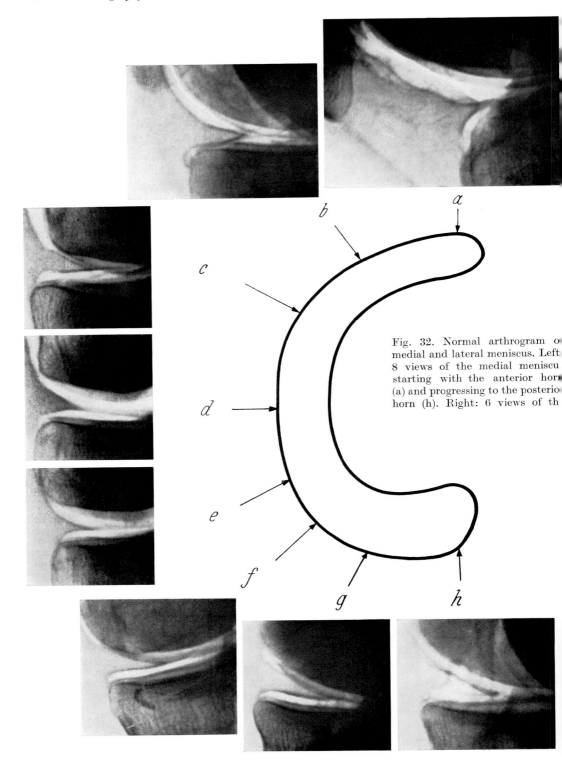

Fig. 32. Normal arthrogram of medial and lateral meniscus. Left 8 views of the medial meniscu starting with the anterior horn (a) and progressing to the posterio horn (h). Right: 6 views of th

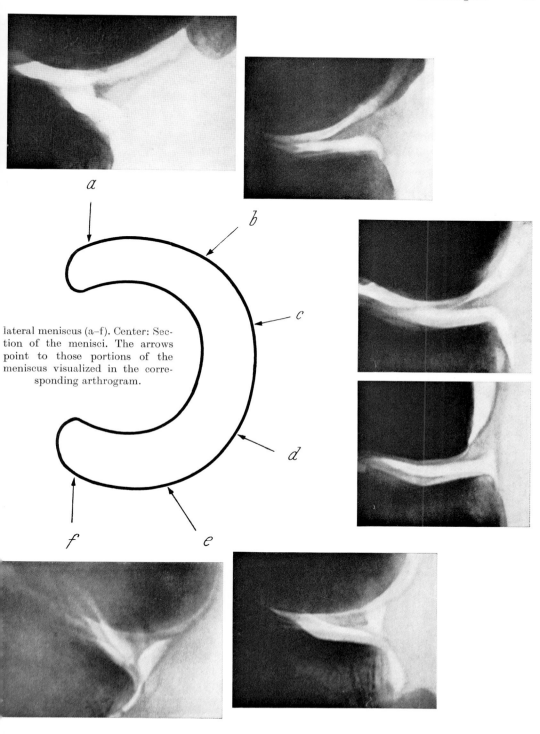

lateral meniscus (a–f). Center: Section of the menisci. The arrows point to those portions of the meniscus visualized in the corresponding arthrogram.

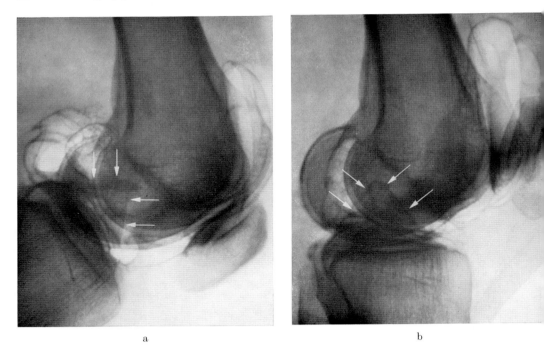

a                                                           b

Fig. 33a and b. Lateral view of the knee joint (double contrast arthrogram) with minimal internal rotation
a) Knee flexed; the cruciate ligaments show sharp contours (arrows). b) Knee extended: the cruciate liga
ments and the articular surface of the patella are well visualized. Both positions give a good view of th
joint spaces.

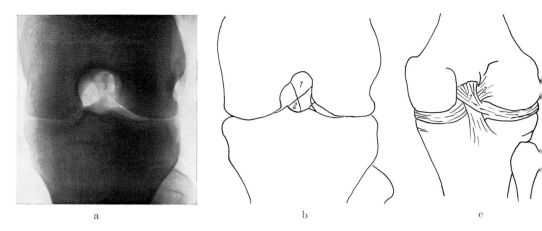

a                                           b                                           c

Fig. 34. AP view of the cruciate ligaments. The knee is flexed 45 degrees. The patient is in a prone positio
a) Arthrogram. b) Drawing: 1. posterior, 2. anterior cruciate ligament, c) corresponding anatomic drawir
(see also Fig. 2).

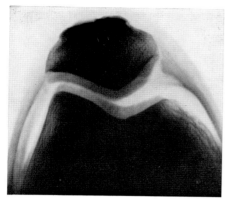

35a

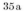

lateral    medial

35b

Fig. 35. Axial view of the patella. a) Arthrogram b) Drawing. Note the sharp contours of the articular cartilage of the patella and its even thickness (arrows).

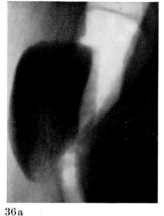

36a                    36b

Fig. 36. Lateral view of the patella with the knee extended. a) Arthrogram. b) Drawing. Note the sharp contours of the patellar articular cartilage (arrows).

never seen a recessus which extended over the entire length of the meniscus. They do not seem to have any pathologic significance but apparently are anatomical fossae. They are shaped like regular, well delineated grooves and can be easily recognized on the arthrogram. Irregular contours or pointed recessus are usually lesions of the meniscus or at least indicate increased mobility of that particular portion of the meniscus.

The cross section of the meniscus varies from one individual to another but also within the same meniscus relative to width and height. According to Lindblom, the average width of the anterior horn of the medial meniscus is

Fig. 37. Articular injection of liquid contrast medium into the loose fatty tissue between the suprapatellar bursa and the anterior surface of the femur. Irregular distribution of contrast medium (arrows).

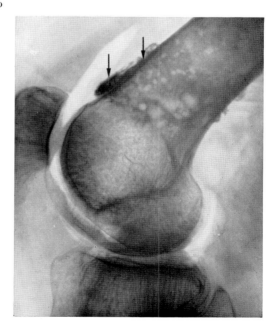

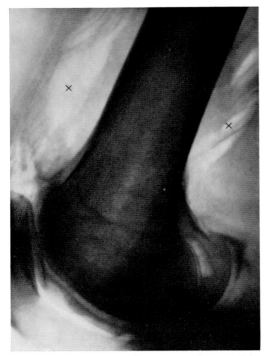

Fig. 38. Periarticular soft tissue emphysema (x).

6 mm., and the posterior horn of the medial meniscus is 14 mm. The anterior horn of the lateral meniscus measures 10 mm. and the posterior horn of the lateral meniscus 9 mm. The height of the menisci is usually 3 to 5 mm. A meniscus which is narrow in one portion is usually narrow in its entire length (Lindblom).

*a) Variations in the Normal Arthrogram of the Medial Meniscus*

The shape of the medial meniscus is different from that of the lateral meniscus. It has the greater curvature and always lies along the edge of the medial tibial plateau. In the arthrogram its capsular attachment blends with the edge of the tibial plateau. Shape and size of the meniscus vary from the anterior horn to the posterior horn. The anterior horn is rather small and short (Fig. 43). Its middle portion is usually of the same size or even smaller; the inner angle is more acute and the femoral and tibial surfaces are often concave (Fig. 44). The posterior horn increases in width and height in the dorsal

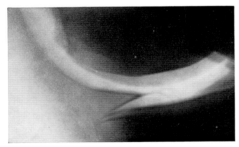
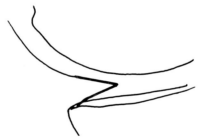

Fig. 39. Arthrogram of a normal meniscus (medial). Wedge-shaped shadow with pointed inner corner. A film of contrast medium increases the contrast. Arthrogram on left, drawing on right.

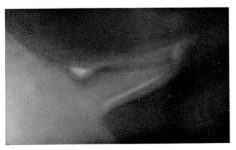
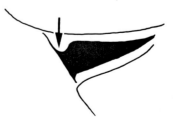

Fig. 40. Normal meniscus (posterior horn, medial meniscus). Arthrogram on left, drawing on right. The recessus between the upper border of the meniscus and the capsule is visualized as a sharply delineated defect (arrow).

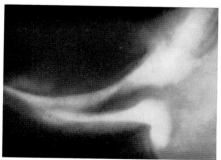 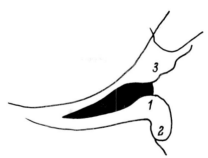

Fig. 41. Normal meniscus (anterior horn of lateral meniscus). Arthrogram on left, drawing on right. 1. Inferior recessus between inferior border of meniscus and capsule. 2. Inferior capsular space. 3. Superior capsular space.

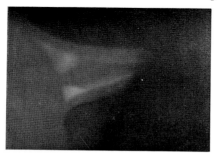 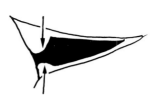

Fig. 42. Normal meniscus (posterior horn of medial meniscus). Superior recessus between superior border of meniscus and joint capsule and inferior recessus between inferior border of meniscus and joint capsule (arrows). (See also Fig. 48.)

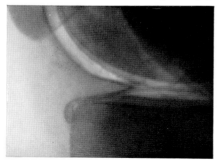 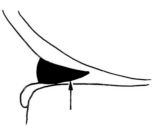

Fig. 43. Normal medial meniscus, anterior horn. Inferior border slightly convex (arrow); average width of the meniscus.

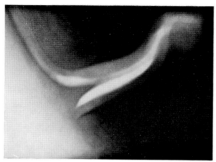 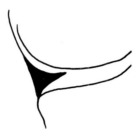

Fig. 44. Normal medial meniscus, middle zone. Cross section of meniscus smaller, contours concave.

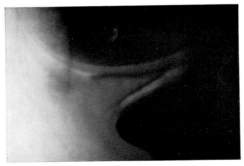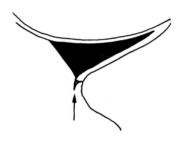

Fig. 45. Normal meniscus, posterior horn. Meniscus wedge much wider and slightly higher than in the area of the anterior horn. The inner border of the wedge is more pointed. The inferior capsular space is visualized as a slot (arrow).

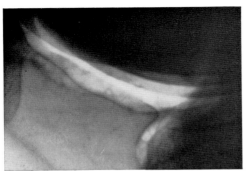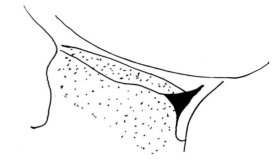

Fig. 46. Normal medial meniscus, anterior horn. Hoffa's fat pad superimposed (dotted area).

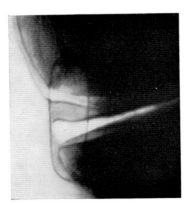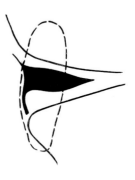

Fig. 47. Normal medial meniscus, posterior horn. Bursa semimembranosogastrocnemica superimposed (interrupted line).

direction and its cross section is a long, pointed wedge (Fig. 45) with a straight tibial surface. The medial meniscus as a whole is shaped like a comma with the posterior horn representing the wide portion of the comma.

Recessus can be found relatively often on the medial side. They are frequently located in the posterior horn area at the junction between the capsule and the meniscus and usually on the femoral surface (Fig. 40). Occasionally they are

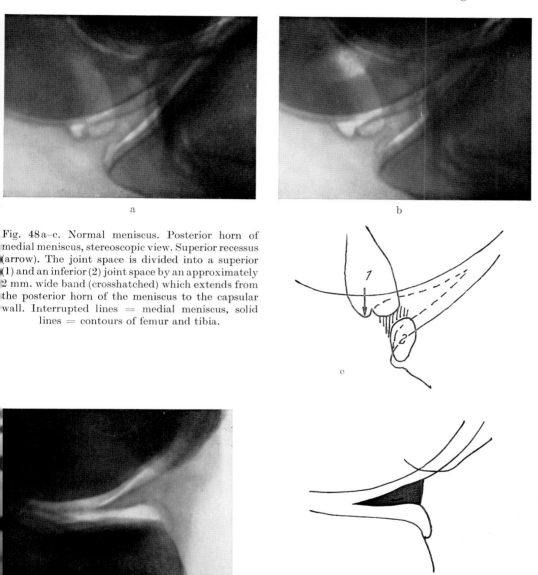

Fig. 48a–c. Normal meniscus. Posterior horn of medial meniscus, stereoscopic view. Superior recessus (arrow). The joint space is divided into a superior (1) and an inferior (2) joint space by an approximately 2 mm. wide band (crosshatched) which extends from the posterior horn of the meniscus to the capsular wall. Interrupted lines = medial meniscus, solid lines = contours of femur and tibia.

Fig. 49. Normal meniscus, anterior horn of lateral meniscus. Wide with pointed inner border.

found on the inferior surface (Fig. 41). Very rarely they may occur on both surfaces simultaneously (Fig. 42). These recessi can be of considerable depth. The picture then resembles a smooth old tear which is covered with synovium and increased mobility of the meniscus must be suspected. The usual diameter of a recessus is approximately 1 to 3 mm. Recessus

are found less frequently in the area of the anterior horn of the medial meniscus. If they occur, they are usually smaller and located on the undersurface.

The anterior horn of the medial meniscus borders on the medial base of the infrapatellar fat pad. Arthrograms in this area can show superimpositions which should not be confused

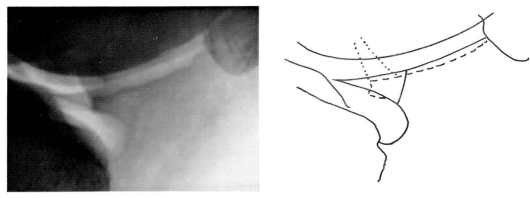

Fig. 50. Lateral meniscus. Hoffa's fat pad (interrupted line) superimposed over anterior portion of anterior horn. Infrapatellar synovial fold (dotted line).

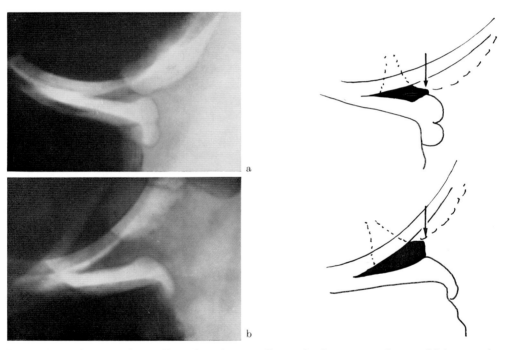

Fig. 51. Normal anterior horn of lateral meniscus. a) Connection between meniscus and joint capsule appears very thin (arrow) = superimposition. b) The same effect less marked. Hoffa's fat pad (interrupted line). Infrapatellar synovial fold (dotted line).

with tears (Fig. 46; see also infrapatellar fat pad).

The bursa semimembranosogastrocnemica frequently is superimposed on the posterior horn of the medial meniscus (see Fig. 47). This, however, does not usually interfere with interpreta-
tion (see also under bursae). The opening of bursa can partially permeate a meniscus (see Fig. 66) or it can develop from a recessus (see Fig. 67). Connection of the meniscus with the capsule is usually fairly tight but can occasionally extend into a narrow tissue bridge toward

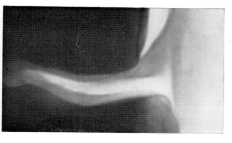
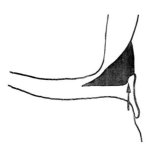

Fig. 52. Middle zone of normal lateral meniscus. Meniscus wedge relatively high. Inferior recessus (arrow).

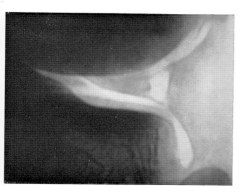
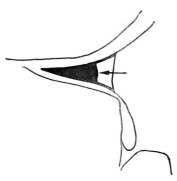

Fig. 53. Posterior horn of normal lateral meniscus interrupted at the junction with the joint capsule by the so-called hiatus popliteus (arrow) except for 2 thin tissue bridges.

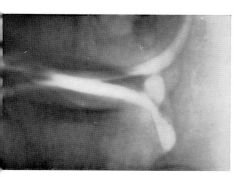
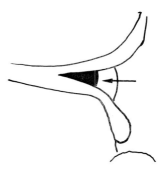

Fig. 54. Posterior horn of lateral meniscus. The tendon sheath of the popliteus muscle (hiatus popliteus) is visualized as a rhomboid structure (arrow).

the end of the posterior horn of the medial meniscus (Rüttimann). This should not be confused with an injury. The tissue bridge presents as two fine slightly curled horziontal lines which are separatedap proximately 1 to 2 mm. They curve to the outside and the upper one blends into the upper and the lower one into the lower edge of the capsule (Fig. 48). These lines gradually disappear towards the inner border of the meniscus. The criteria for these findings are so clear-cut that the correct interpretation should not present any difficulties. It is possible, however, that these posterior horns are more prone to dislocation or tear.

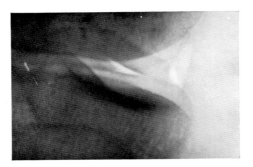 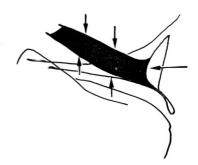

Fig. 55. Posterior horn of lateral meniscus at the hiatus popliteus slightly more dorsal than Fig. 53. Hiatus popliteus more oval-shaped (horizontal arrow). Note the posterior horn of the lateral meniscus (vertical arrow) which is seen as a band-like shadow and rises slightly towards the interior of the joint (black).

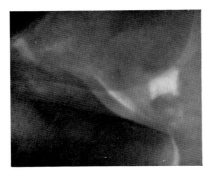 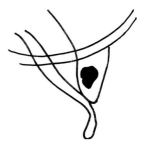

Fig. 56. Tendon sheath of the popliteus which surrounds the tendon completely. The tendon is visualized in cross section (black).

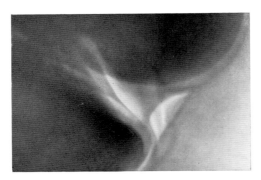 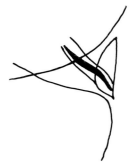

Fig. 57. Tendon of the popliteus muscle (black) running obliquely within the tendon sheath.

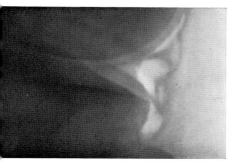 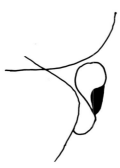

Fig. 58. Tendon of the popliteus muscle (black) alongside the outer wall of the hiatus.

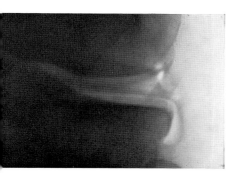 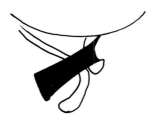

ig. 59. Tendon of the popliteus muscle (black) projected across the hiatus. (Position approximately one cm. more ventral than that in Fig. 57.)

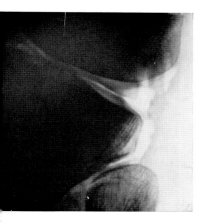 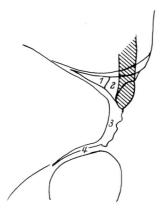

ig. 60. Demonstration of structures in the area of the posterior horn of the lateral meniscus. 1. Posterior orn. 2. Tendon sheath of the popliteus tendon. 3. Inferior capsular space connected with popliteus tendon sheath. 4. Tibial-fibular joint, crosshatched=popliteus tendon.

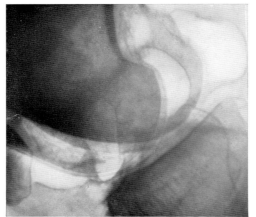

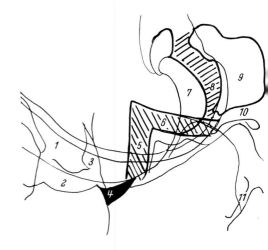

Fig. 61. Demonstration of the anterior and the posterior portion of the divided joint space. Lateral view in slight internal rotation: 1. Anterior joint space, 2. Hoffa's fat pad, 3. Infrapatellar synovial fold, 4. Lateral meniscus, 5. Anterior cruciate ligament, 6. Posterior cruciate ligament, 7. Lateral portion of the posterior joint space, 8. Posterior sagittal capsular fold with fat pad, 9. Medial aspect of the posterior joint space, 10. Medial meniscus, posterior horn, 11. Tibial-fibular joint.

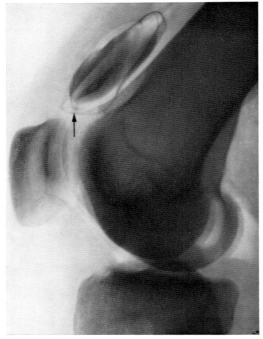

Fig. 62. Suprapatellar pouch (filled with air and liquid contrast medium) completely separated from the remaining joint space (filled with air) by a septum (arrow).

## b) Variations of the Normal Lateral Meniscus

The lateral meniscus differs from the media in that the radius of its curvature is smaller. I usually represents an almost closed ring. It width changes little between the anterior an the posterior horn. According to Lindblom th average width of the anterior horn is 10 mm whereas that of the posterior horn is 9 mm. Th anterior horn has a rather long, pointed inne border (Figs. 49 and 50). A tissue bridge connect it with the joint capsule.

The infrapatellar fat pad can be superimpose on the anterior horn of the lateral meniscus i an arthrogram of this area. This, however, i less likely to lead to misinterpretation becaus the anterior horn of the lateral meniscus is large than that of the medial. It extends further int the joint, and can be delineated more readi (Fig. 51). The tissue bridge between the anteri horn of the lateral meniscus and the capsule ca occasionally appear rather thin, but this appear ance is usually produced by superimposition the infrapatellar fat pad.

Occasionally a recessus is found on the unde surface of the anterior horn of the lateral meni cus or the tissue bridge between the capsule an the meniscus (Fig. 52). This recessus is relativel narrow and long. Accessory bursae are rare o the lateral side.

The middle zone of the lateral meniscu shows a typical cross section which makes i easily recognizable. The base of the wedge a

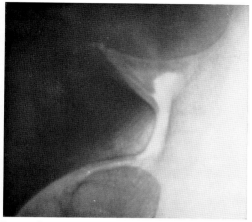
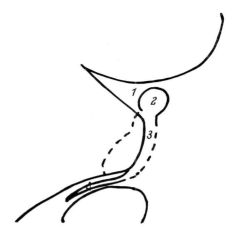

Fig. 63. Popliteal bursa. 1. Lateral meniscus, posterior horn. 2. Hiatus popliteus. 3. Popliteal bursa (interrupted line) and inferior capsular space. 4. Tibial-fibular joint.

ts capsular attachments is relatively high. A recessus is usually situated at the inferior capsular attachment and continues dorsally into the popliteus tendon sheath of the posterior horn Fig. 53). The junction of the posterior horn of the lateral meniscus with the capsule is interrupted by the tendon sheath of the popliteus muscle (hiatus popliteus) (Fig. 54). The appearance of the hiatus popliteus is typical and should not be misinterpreted:

1) Typical location in the posterior horn of the lateral meniscus.

2) It is smooth and sharply delineated.

3) It is slot-shaped in appearance. The slot can vary from triangular to oval (Fig. 55).

4) The popliteus tendon can occasionally be visualized either as a band of approximately 2 to 5 mm. in thickness which runs in an oblique direction from caudal to cranial as an indentation in the lateral wall of the hiatus or as a round shadow if the tendon is surrounded entirely by the tendon sheath (less frequent) (Fig. 56). Unfortunately the popliteus tendon cannot always be seen (Figs. 57 to 60) because the tendon sheath surrounds only a small portion of the tendon. If the tendon cannot be visualized it does not necessarily mean that it is torn or was cut during surgery. Several authors have expressed the opinion that the action of the popliteus muscle as a tensor of the capsule is important and that its removal leads to symptoms.

## 2) Joint Spaces and Joint Capsule

The embryonal knee joint is divided into a superior and an inferior capsular space by a horizontal septum. The menisci later develop from the border of this septum. The infrapatellar fat pad with its plica synovialis infrapatellaris, the posterior fat pad, the cruciate ligaments and their synovial covering are remnants of an embryonal sagittal septum and separate the medial from the lateral joint space.

In the adult individual we can also differentiate a superior and an inferior *capsular space* which are separated by the attachment of the meniscus to the joint capsule (see Fig. 41). The synovial membrane does not cover the menisci and is thus also interrupted. The inferior capsular space varies considerably. On the medial side it is usually larger anteriorly than posteriorly, where it is frequently only a small slot (see Figs. 43, 45). On the lateral side the inferior capsular space can be quite large anteriorly (Fig. 41) while posteriorly its size varies. Occasionally this space is fairly wide and is connected with the tendon sheath of the popliteus tendon, thus connecting the knee joint with the tibiofibular joint (Fig. 60).

The vertical division of the posterior joint space can be demonstrated quite well in the arthrogram with the knee in slight flexion and rotation. (Fig. 61). The dorsally convex contour

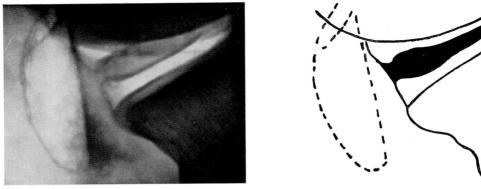

Fig. 64. Bursa semimembranosogastrocnemica (interrupted line) seen outside the posterior horn of the medial meniscus.

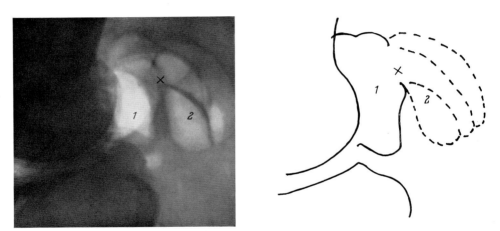

Fig. 65. Bursa semimembranosogastrocnemica at broad entrance to the bursa in the upper portion of the posterior wall of the medial portion of the posterior joint space. 1. Posterior joint space, 2. Bursa (interrupted line), x) Entrance to the bursa. The bursa is loculated.

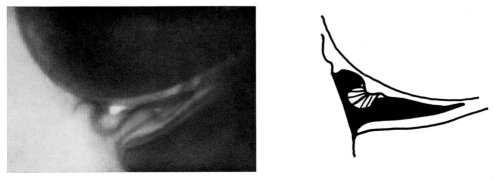

Fig. 66. Medial mensicus, posterior horn. Entrance to the bursa (crosshatched) crosses the upper surface of the meniscus.

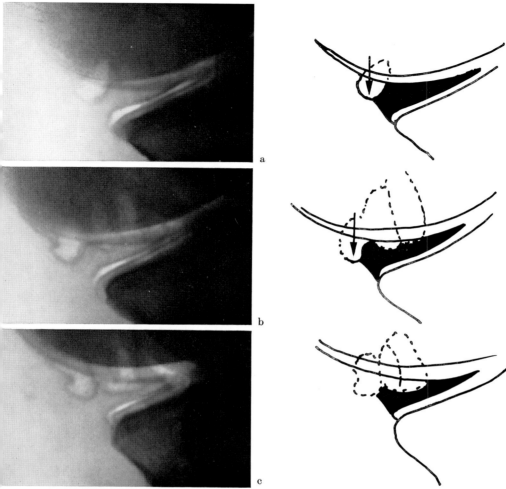

Fig. 67. Medial meniscus, posterior horn. a) Central portion of the posterior horn, b) one exposure and c) two exposures farther posteriorly. The recussus-like structure in the superior capsular attachment at (a) continues on into a bursa in (b) and (c) (interrupted line).

of the posterior sagittal capsular fold is typical and indentations from pathologic processes are quite obvious (see Fig. 203).

The *superior recessus* (suprapatellar pouch) is described in the section on bursae (see below).

The *joint capsule* is covered evenly with synovial membrane and has a smooth sharply delineated appearance in the arthrogram (see Fig. 61). The so-called central joint space is not accurately localized anatomically and arthrographically. It comprises the intercondylar area of the tibia and the intercondylar fossa of the femur, the space and soft tissues between them

and the neighboring articular surfaces of the tibia. This central joint space is difficult to evaluate in the arthrogram because of its hidden location. Pathologic changes in it are difficult to visualize. Its irregular shape can, for instance, cause loose bodies or meniscus fragments to "disappear" in it. In these cases the diagnosis must be made from other arthrographic signs.

## 3) Bursae

The knee joint is connected with several bursae. The most important of these is the

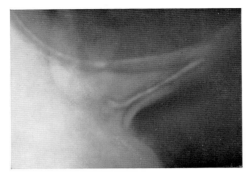 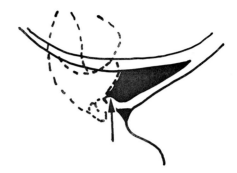

Fig. 68. Entrance into the bursa semimembranosogastrocnemica (interrupted line). The entrance begins a so-called inferior recessus (arrow) at the posterior horn of the medial meniscus.

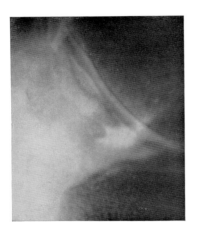 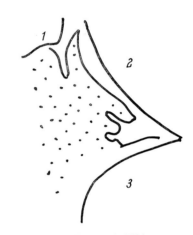

Fig. 69. Infrapatellar fat pad (dotted), villous. 1. Patella. 2. Femur. 3. Tibia.

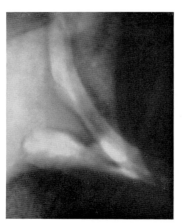 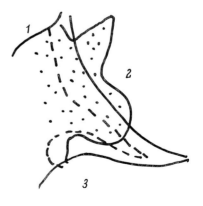

Fig. 70. Infrapatellar fat pad (dotted). Lateral view with slight internal rotation. 1. Patella, 2. Femur, 3. Tib (interrupted line): the capsular wall continues laterally and caudally into the lateral meniscus adjacent to t fat pad.

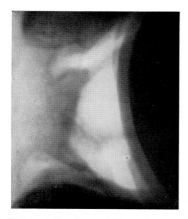

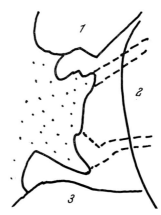

Fig. 71. Infrapatellar fat pad (dotted) with a double infrapatellar synovial fold (interrupted line). 1. Patella. 2. Femur. 3. Tibia.

*bursa suprapatellaris* (superior recessus, suprapatellar pouch). In the fetus it develops as the bursa subtendinea of the quadriceps muscle and is completely separated from the knee joint. The connection with the joint is established shortly before birth. This connection is frequently incomplete and remnants of a septum can often be recognized. In rare cases the suprapatellar pouch can remain completely separated from the knee joint. Injection of liquid contrast medium into the completely separated suprapatellar pouch represents a typical picture (see Fig. 62). The effective size of the bursa varies. In the adult it extends approximately 7 cm. proximal to the proximal border of the patella. On the ventral side the synovial lining of the bursa is intimately connected with the posterior surface of the quadriceps femoris. Its dorsal layer is separated from the anterior surface of the femur by a loose, fatty tissue. Periarticular deposits of contrast medium are occasionally injected into this area because resistance to injection is minimal and the examiner may be deceived about the position of his needle (see Fig. 37).

The *bursa poplitea* is located between the posterior surface of the tibia and the popliteal muscle (Fig. 63). It is frequently connected with the knee joint through the tendon sheath of the popliteus muscle and can also have a direct connection with the tibiofibular joint.

*Bursa semimembranosogastrocnemica*

The tibial head of the gastrocnemius muscle arises proximally from the tibial condyle of the femur and the joint capsule. The bursa is located under its origin. The semimembranosus muscle, which attaches on the medial side of the proximal tibia, forms a bursa where it crosses the tibial head of the gastrocnemius. The bursae of these two muscles quite frequently join to form one bursa which is connected with the joint (Fig. 64). In the arthrogram it is superimposed over the posterior horn of the medial meniscus (see Fig. 47). The openings to these bursae can often be visualized quite well. A high orifice (of the bursa gastrocnemica) can sometimes be seen quite well in the lateral view of the arthrogram. It is located in the upper half of the posteromedial joint space (Fig. 65). If the entrance to the bursa semimembranosa is located more distally, it can perforate the posterior horn of the medial meniscus on its superior or inferior surface. It can then resemble a recessus (Figs. 66–68). Small accessory bursae can occasionally be seen. Brantigan and Voshell have found bursae between the medial meniscus and the medial collateral ligament. According to Lindblom these bursae are always pathologic. In his autopsy material he found them only in those cases where a tear of the meniscus was present. Our own experience agrees with Lindblom's findings.

### 4) The Infrapatellar Fat Pad

The infrapatellar fat pad is a fatty cushion on the dorsal side of the ligamentum patellae proprium and is covered by synovial membrane. It is of cylindrical shape and fills the space between femur, tibia and cruciate ligaments when the knee is flexed (see Fig. 4).

On the lateral view of the arthrogram the infrapatellar fat pad often shows irregular, relatively flat contours (see Fig. 46). Occasionally it may show a villous surface (Fig. 69). The basal portions are usually superimposed on the anterior horns of the menisci (Figs. 46, 50 and 70).

The remnant of the embryonal sagittal fold often forms a plica synovialis infrapatellaris (see Fig. 50) which extends from the infrapatellar fat pad through the anterior joint space to the distal edge of the intercondylar fossa of the femur. It can be recognized in all its variants in the lateral arthrogram. Rarely it can be double (Fig. 71). Course and position of the plica change with increased flexion of the knee because of the displacement of its insertion in the intercondylar fossa. Since no normal values have been established, the size of the infrapatellar fat pad is difficult to evaluate. So-called hypertrophies or hemorrhages are difficult to diagnose. So far we have not been able to establish such a diagnosis in our own material. Occasionally we have suspected this condition from arthrographic findings which were later confirmed at surgery.

### 5) The Dorsal Fat Pad

The dorsal fat pad is located in the synovial fold which extends from the dorsal capsule ventrally covering both cruciate ligaments and dividing the posterior joint space sagittally into two halves. It can be visualized on rotation views of the posterior joint space (see Fig. 61). Calcifications of the posterior fat pad are relatively frequent.

### 6) The Cruciate Ligaments

The cruciate ligaments are located in the intercondylar area. They are completely covered by synovial membrane which makes their local

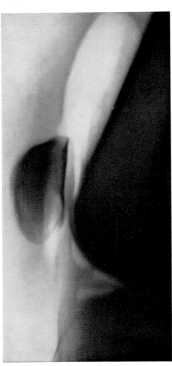
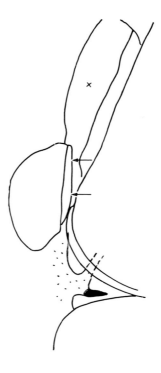

Fig. 72. Articular surface of the patella in the lateral tomogram. Arthrogram done with air only; note Hoffa's fat pad (dotted) with infrapatellar synovial fold (interrupted line) and the lateral meniscus (anterior horn, black). x) suprapatellar pouch.

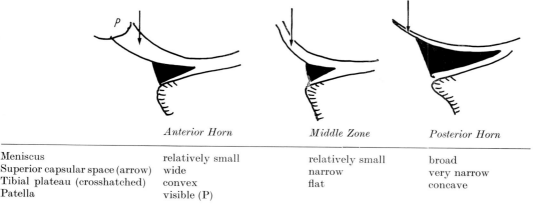

| | *Anterior Horn* | *Middle Zone* | *Posterior Horn* |
|---|---|---|---|
| Meniscus | relatively small | relatively small | broad |
| Superior capsular space (arrow) | wide | narrow | very narrow |
| Tibial plateau (crosshatched) | convex | flat | concave |
| Patella | visible (P) | | |

Fig. 73. *Medial meniscus.* Localizing signs.

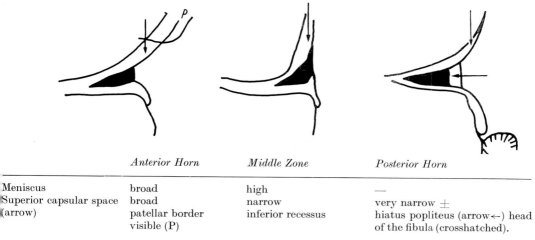

| | *Anterior Horn* | *Middle Zone* | *Posterior Horn* |
|---|---|---|---|
| Meniscus | broad | high | — |
| Superior capsular space (arrow) | broad | narrow | very narrow ± |
| | patellar border visible (P) | inferior recessus | hiatus popliteus (arrow←) head of the fibula (crosshatched). |

Fig. 74. *Lateral Meniscus.* Localizing signs.

tion extracapsular. They serve as axial stabilizers of the knee (Toendury) and cross inside the joint. The anterior cruciate ligament arises in the anterior intercondylar area between the anterior attachments of the menisci and stretches obliquely to the inner surface of the lateral femoral condyle posteriorly. Occasionally additional ligamentous bands go from the anterior cruciate ligament into the intercondylar fossa and even to the medial femoral condyle (Lindblom). The posterior cruciate ligament arises in the posterior intercondylar area of the tibia behind the attachments of the posterior horns of the menisci and extends in an oblique direction to the inside of the medial femoral condyle anteriorly. Both cruciate ligaments can be differentiated well in the lateral view of the arthrogram with slight internal rotation (see Fig. 33). The anterior cruciate ligament can be visualized on spot views of the anterior horn of the medial meniscus, the posterior cruciate on spot views of both posterior horns. Their contours in the lateral view form a tent-shaped, sharply delineated shadow over the tibial spines. The anterior double contour represents the anterior, the posterior double contour the posterior cruciate (Fig. 61). The cruciate ligaments can also be visualized quite well in the anterior posterior view (see Fig. 34).

## 7) Articular Surfaces

Both *femoral condyles* have the shape of a cylinder and are separated by the intercondylar fossa. Their cartilaginous surface can be visualized in the arthrogram quite well as a regular, smooth cover which is slightly more dense than the soft tissue shadow and less dense than the bony shadow (see Fig. 39).

The articular surface of the *tibia* is a single large plateau. We distinguish two condylar fossae which are slightly concave and are covered by cartilage. They are separated by the intercondylar area which is not covered with cartilage. The cartilaginous surfaces of the tibia can be differentiated quite well in the arthrogram see Fig. 52).

The articular surface of the *patella* protrudes like a flat roof with a smaller medial and a larger lateral portion. Its cartilaginous covering can be visualized in the lateral and the axial view of the arthrogram (Figs. 35–36). Pathologic changes in the articular cartilage of the patella can occasionally be demonstrated. Tomograms combined with double contrast arthrography increase the diagnostic possibilities (Fuermaier) (Figs. 72, 191).

## 8) Anatomical Characteristics of Different Meniscus Segments in Serial Views

We usually arrange our multiple spot views in such a manner that their sequence from the upper left-hand to the lower right-hand corner represents the entire course of the meniscus from the anterior to the posterior horn. The first views represent the anterior, the last views the posterior horn, Knowledge of the anatomic

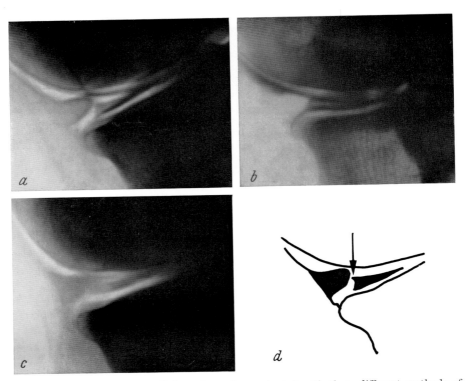

Fig. 75. Vertical tear of the same medial meniscus demonstrated with three different methods of arthrography: a) Double contrast method. b) Positive contrast (with contrast medium alone). c) Negative contrast (air arthrogram). d) Drawing for (a) to (c). Meniscus black. The arrow points to the tear.

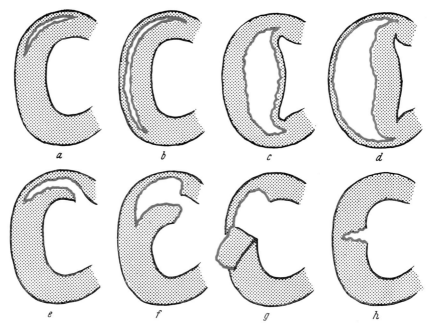

Fig. 76. (= 15) Schematic drawing of the most frequent meniscus injuries. a–d) Longitudinal tears. c, d) Total tear with dislocation of the inner fragment into the joint (so-called bucket handle tears). a, b) Partial longitudinal tears. e–g) Mixed forms: unilateral tears of fragments with and without displacement. h) Transverse tear.

characteristics of different meniscus segments and their surroundings permits fairly accurate localization of a meniscus segment in one single view. These characteristics are summarized in figures 73 and 74.

# E. The Abnormal Arthrogram

## 1) Meniscus Injuries

The double contrast method is especially suitable for demonstration of meniscus injuries. It combines the advantages of pure air arthrography – good visualization of the internal structures of the knee because of extension of the joint capsule from the air – with those of arthrography with a positive contrast medium – such as good contrast and sharp contours. A tear in the meniscus (Fig. 75) shows up as an air-filled slot which is delineated from the soft tissue shadow of the meniscus by a thin film of contrast medium. The double contrast arthrogram

produces a greater difference in density, namely, between contrast medium and air, than each of the two methods alone where we have contrast between dye and tissues or between tissues and air.

The drawings in Fig. 76 show the more common meniscus lesions. We can distinguish the following meniscus tears:

*1) Longitudinal tears:*

a) Simple longitudinal tears, partial or total (Figs. 76a–76d, 77);

b) Complex longitudinal tears with dislocation of the inner fragment (bucket-handle tear) (Figs. 76c, d, 78–80).

*2) Transverse tears* (Figs. 76h, 81).

*3) Complex tears* (mixed forms) (Figs. 82–84) (e.g. unilateral detachment of fragments with or without displacement).

*4) Total detachment* (detachment from the capsule, disinsertion) (Fig. 85).

Fig. 77. Partial longitudinal tear of the medial meniscus (posterior horn). *Above:* Schematic drawing: Left: meniscus cross sections in black. a) Anterior horn intact. b) Posterior horn with tear (arrow) close to the inner border. Right: Drawing of the entire meniscus, (tear = wavy lines). *Below:* Similar case. Left: Arthrograms. a) Anterior horn. b) Posterior horn. Right: Surgical specimen.

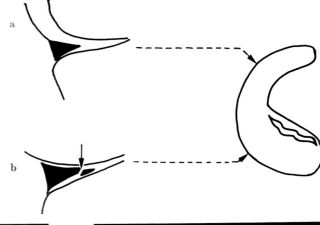

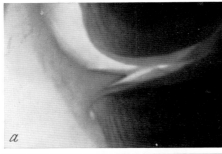

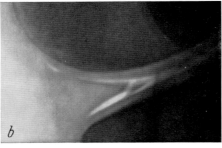

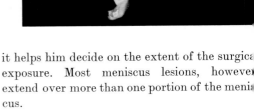

All forms and directions of tears can occur in all portions of the meniscus, as single or as multiple tears. In the arthrogram we can see only a cross section of the meniscus and we differentiate the following meniscus tears: a) vertical tears (Figs. 86–89); b) oblique tears (concentric tears) (Figs. 90–94); horizontal tears (Figs. 95–99); d) mixed forms (Fig. 100–102).

Meniscus lesions can be classified as anterior horn tears, central tears or posterior horn tears but only when the tears are less extensive such as transverse tears. Exact localization of the tear can be important for the surgeon because

it helps him decide on the extent of the surgical exposure. Most meniscus lesions, however, extend over more than one portion of the meniscus.

Studies on the *frequency* of different meniscus lesions, as far as their *location* is concerned, have produced the following results: The medial meniscus is injured much more frequently than the lateral due to its firm attachment to the medial collateral ligament. Its posterior horn is injured most often with tears on the inferior surface being more frequent than those on the superior surface (Lindblom). Injuries in the middle zone are less frequent and injuries to the anterior horn are even more rare. Lesions in the lateral meniscus, on the other hand, are more frequently located in the anterior horn.

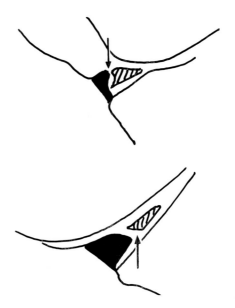

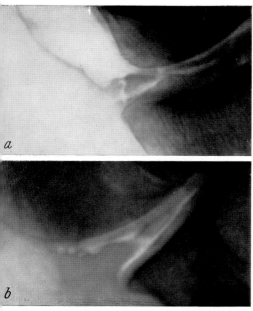

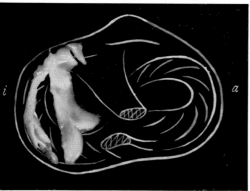

Fig. 78. Subtotal longitudinal tear without marked displacement of the inner fragment.
*Above:* Left: Arthrograms. a) Anterior horn. b) Posterior horn. Right: Drawing: The displacement of the inner fragment (crosshatched) measures 2 to 3 mm.
*Below:* Surgical specimen: Subtotal longitudinal tear of the mediai meniscus. Displacement of fragments is somewhat more than seen on the arthrogram.

## b) Longitudinal Tears

The longitudinal tear is the most frequent form of meniscus injury. It can be visualized very clearly in the arthrogram because it runs in an orthograde direction with the X-ray beam (see Fig. 29). It can present itself in the cross section as a vertical, an oblique (concentric) or horizontal tear, or it can vary in its direction. The different forms of longitudinal tears are demonstrated in Figs. 77–80. In most buckethandle tears even the transition from the bucket to the handle can be seen in the anterior and posterior horns (Figs. 79–80).

A totally detached fragment can occasionally be resorbed completely. The diagnosis must then be made from a thorough analysis of the stump. The defect in the stump originally represents a negative of the torn fragment. Degenerative and regenerative changes will, however, gradually change its shape. Regenerative changes occur most likely in tears close to the capsule in the so-called regenerative zone of the meniscus. Mechanical effects on the stump will gradually change its shape into that of a wedge which occasionally can resemble the cross section of a normal meniscus.

The *direction* of a meniscus tear in the cross section can show a number of variations: Vertical tears are usually close to the capsule like the so-called disinsertion (complete detachment). They are also found in the middle portion or toward the inner border (Figs. 86–89).

*Oblique tears* (concentric tears) can be found in many different variations and can originate

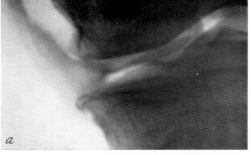

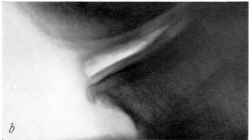

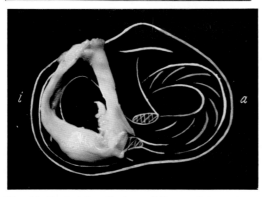

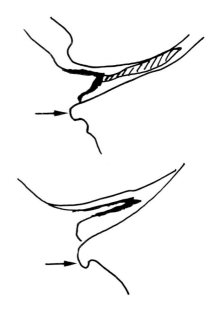

Fig. 79. Bucket handle tear of the medial meniscus. *Above:* Arthrograms with drawings. a) Anterior horn. b) Posterior horn. The displaced fragment (crosshatched), and the stump near the capsule are soaked with contrast medium (thickened black contours). This is a sign of degenerative change. The connection between the stump and the fragment is visible in the area of the anterior horn. Note the severe secondary arthrosis with spur formation on the tibial plateau (arrow) in a 32-year-old male. *Below:* Surgical specimen.

from either the superior or inferior surface (Figs. 90–94).

*Horizontal tears* are more frequent in the lateral meniscus but can also occur on the medial side. Dysplastic menisci have a tendency to tear horizontally (Figs. 95–99).

*Mixed forms:* horizontal, oblique and vertical injuries can have angular (Figs. 100 and 101) or stellate shape (Fig. 102).

The *extent* of a meniscus injury can be very small. Small and minimal tears, especially on the inferior surface of the posterior horn, are not infrequent (Figs. 103–106). Severe injuries lead to destructive changes and defects (Figs. 107 to 117), ragged appearance (Figs. 118–121), or fragmentation (Figs. 122–128).

### b) Transverse Tears

Transverse tears can be overlooked very easily with any method of arthrography because the meniscus tear is not orthograde but vertical to the direction of the X-ray beam. It comprises only a short segment of the entire length of the meniscus, and we can find intact meniscus anteriorly and posteriorly to the injured segment (see Fig. 81, upper right). Even with a relatively large number of spot views we cannot always be sure that we have not missed a transverse tear. A pure transverse tear, however, is relatively rare. Usually it is combined with a short longitudinal tear which makes arthrographic diagnosis easier. A certain blurriness of contour or a decrease of contrast density in the arthro-

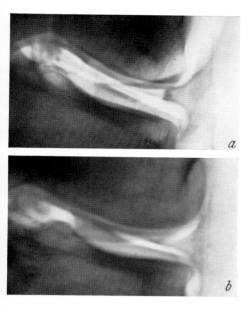

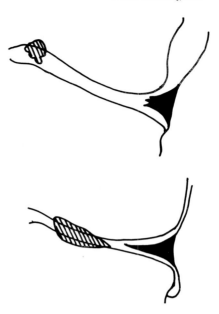

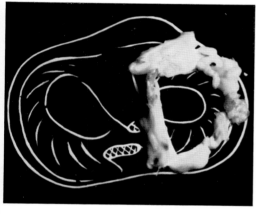

Fig. 80. Bucket handle tear of the lateral meniscus. *Above:* Left: Arthrograms. a) Anterior horn. b) Posterior horn. Right: The corresponding drawings. The fragment that is displaced into the joint (crosshatched) corresponds to the "handle of the bucket." *Below:* Surgical specimen.

gram of the inner portion of the meniscus should make one suspicious of a transverse tear. The tear is frequently delineated on the outer side by a sharp line of contrast which permeates the cross section of the meniscus in a vertical or oblique direction (Fig. 81 b). Obvious overlapping of two wedge-shaped shadows is also a suspicious but not a certain sign.

#### c) Complex Tears (Mixed Forms)

These are formed by a combination of longitudinal and transverse tears. They can lead to single or multiple detachments with or without dislocation of the free fragment. The arthrogram and also the surgical specimen of the injured meniscus show varying and sometimes bizarre forms of complex tears (Figs. 82–84, 100–102).

#### d) Complete Detachment (Disinsertion)

Complete detachment of the meniscus usually produces unequivocal clinical findings, and the patient is usually taken to surgery without an arthrogram. Capsular detachment of the meniscus can be clearly visualized in the arthrogram (Fig. 85).

Occasionally it is possible to determine the *age of a meniscus lesion* radiographically (Lindblom, Rauber). This is made possible by certain direct signs on the meniscus proper and indirect signs on the adjacent cartilage and bone. Routine X-ray views and arthrograms complement each other.

*Direct signs*

The arthrogram of a fresh meniscus lesion shows sharp contours. An old injury, on the other hand, shows completely smooth borders

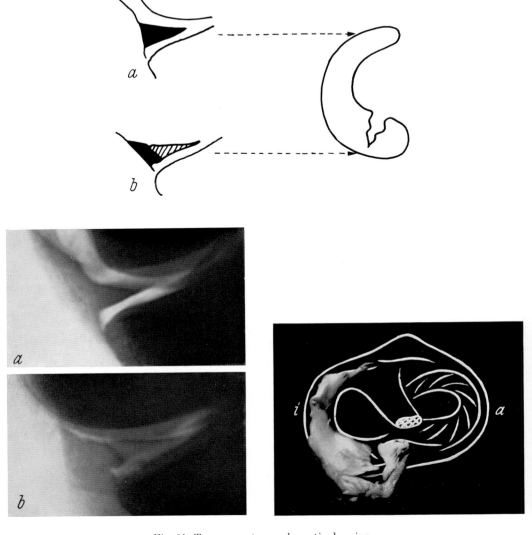

Fig. 81. Transverse tear, schematic drawing.

*Above:* Left: cross sections of the meniscus. a) Anterior horn intact. b) Posterior horn with transverse tear: the tear does not go through the entire width of the meniscus but leaves a small outer portion undamaged (black stump). The inner, less dense portion (crosshatched) shows a wedge-shaped form despite the tear because the intact portions adjacent to the tear are projected over it. The extent of the meniscus tear is shown by the inner vertical border of the stump (black).

*Below:* Similar case. Left: arthrogram of the anterior horn (a) and the posterior horn (b). Right: corresponding surgical specimen.

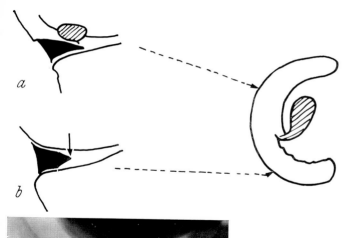

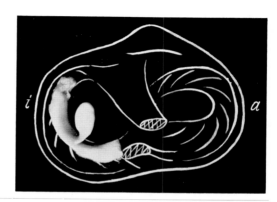

Fig. 82. Complex tear. Longitudinal tear with unilateral tear of the medial posterior horn and displacement of the fragment into the joint.

*Above:* Schematic drawing. Left: cross sections of the meniscus. a) Anterior horn intact (black), displaced fragment (crosshatched). b) Posterior horn with blunted inner border = tear. Right: schematic drawing of the meniscus, displaced fragment (crosshatched), wavy line = tear.

*Below:* Similar case. Left: Arthrogram. a) Anterior horn. b) Posterior horn. Right: corresponding surgical specimen.

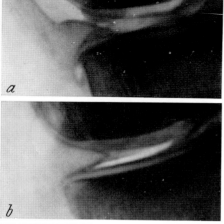

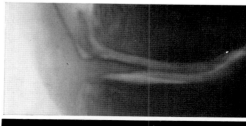

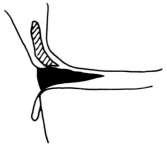

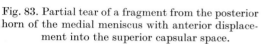

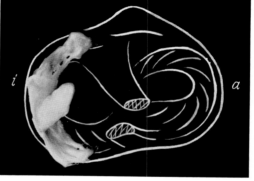

Fig. 83. Partial tear of a fragment from the posterior horn of the medial meniscus with anterior displacement into the superior capsular space.

Right: Above: arthrogram of the meniscus at the junction between the anterior horn and the middle segments.

Left: Drawing: The fragment (crosshatched) is located in the superior capsular space. Meniscus black.

Right: Surgical specimen of the same case. The fragment is torn off the posterior horn and displaced anteriorly.

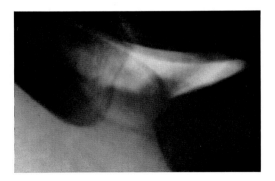

Fig. 84. Partial tear with displacement of the meniscus fragment into the anterior superior capsular space. Left: above, arthrogram of the anterior horn. Below: corresponding drawing. The fragment (crosshatched) is displaced almost vertically. 1. Patella. 2. Femur. 3. Tibia. Right: Surgical specimen. The anterior horn of the meniscus is torn at the junction with the middle zone and displaced upward and anteriorly.

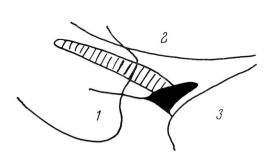

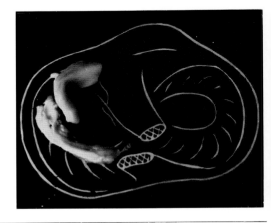

Fig. 85. Total separation of the medial meniscus without displacement. Left: Above, arthrogram of the middle zone: Below, corresponding drawing. The meniscus (black) is torn vertically near the capsule (arrow). The tear is one mm. wide. Right: Surgical specimen. Note the smooth outer surface (= tear) of the meniscus. Additional finding: small transverse tear.

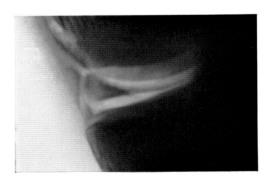

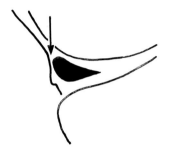

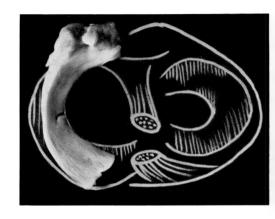

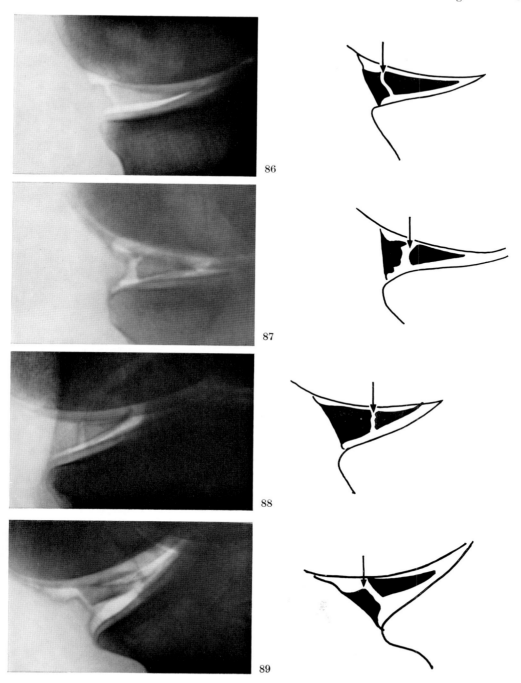

Figs. 86–89. *Vertical tears*. The arrow in the drawing points to the tear. Figs. 86, 87: Tears close to the capsule. 88: Tear in the middle of the meniscus. 89: Tear close to the capsule with slight displacement of the inner fragment in a cranial direction.

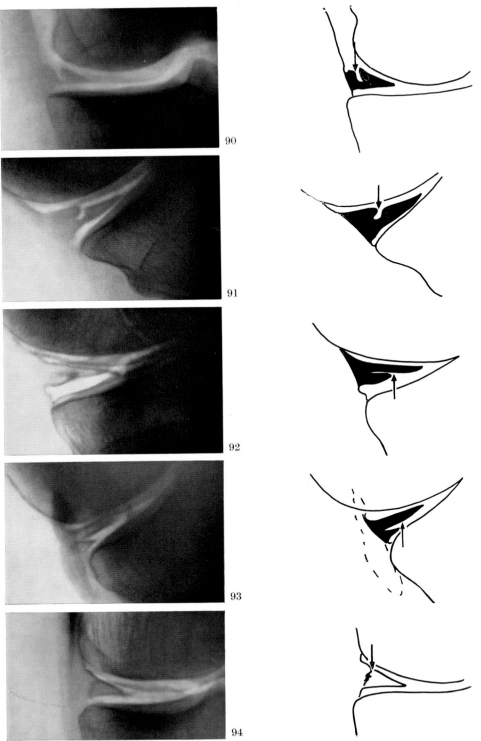

Figs. 90–94. *Oblique tears* (= concentric tears). The arrow in the drawing points to the tear. 90, 91: Tear in the superior surface of the meniscus. 92. 93: Tear in the inferior surface of the meniscus. 94: Complete oblique tear stained with contrast medium.

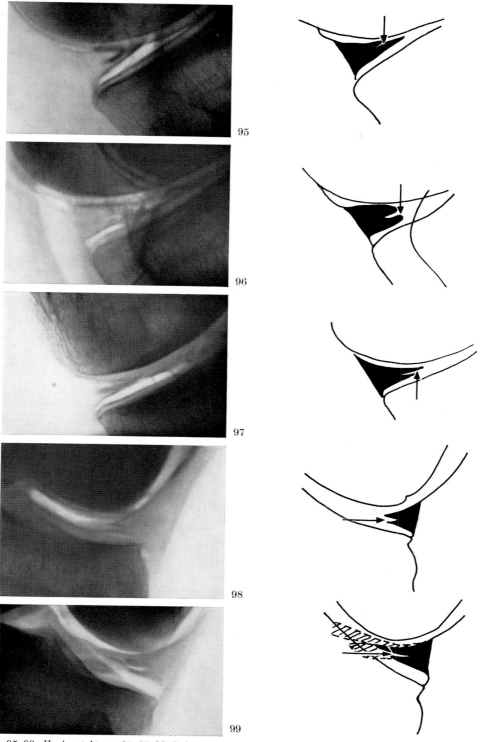

Figs. 95–99. *Horizontal tears*. 95–97: Medial. 98, 99: Lateral. 95, 96: Tear in the superior surface of the posterior horn. 97: Tear in the inferior surface of the meniscus. 98, 99: Tear in the inner border of the anterior horn of the lateral meniscus.

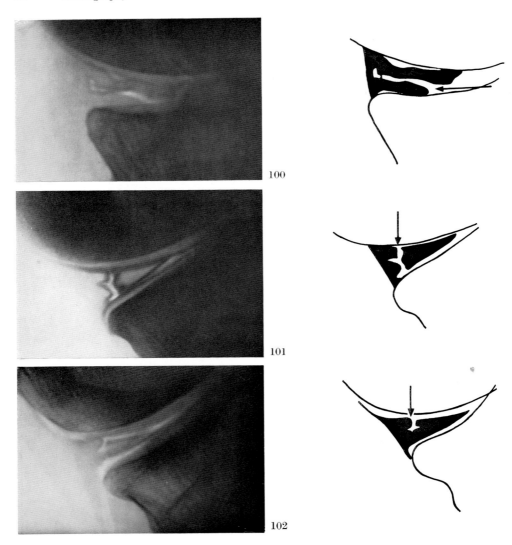

Figs. 100–102: *Mixed forms* (combinations of vertical, horizontal, and oblique tears). 100: Almost horizontal tear with angulation in a cranial direction near the capsule. 101: Y-shaped tear. 102: Stellate tear.

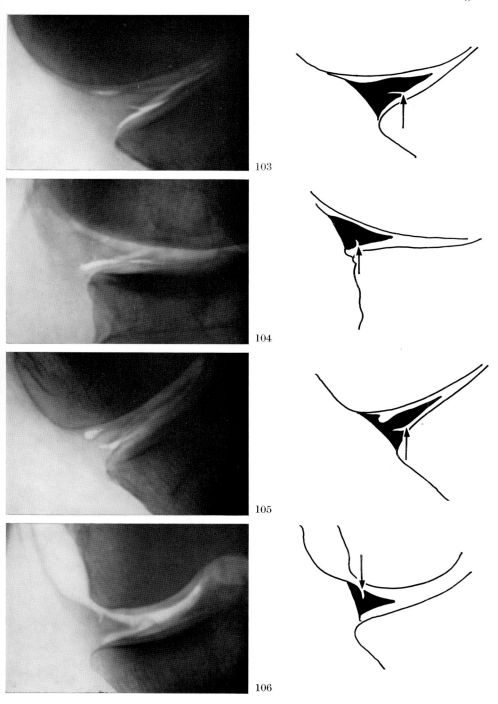

Figs. 103–106. *Small incomplete tears.* 103–105: On the inferior surface of the meniscus (posterior horn of the medial meniscus). 106: Tear on the superior surface of the meniscus close to the capsule.

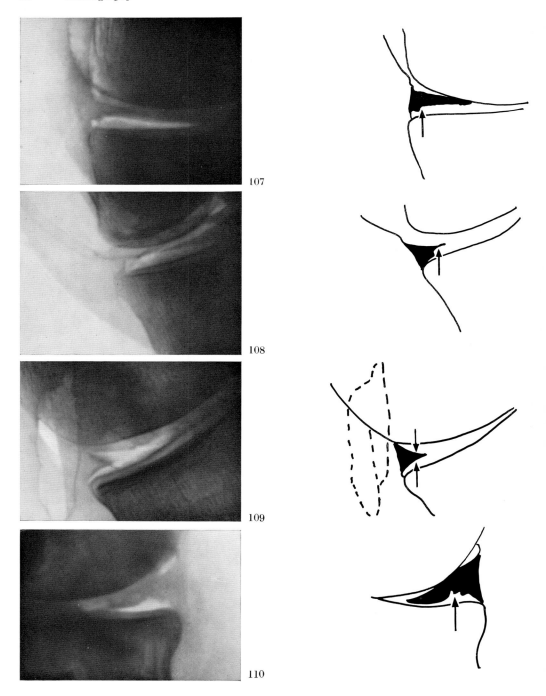

Figs. 107–110. *Meniscus defects*. Torn fragments are not visualized in the joint. Arrows point to the defect 107, 108: Small step formation on the inferior surface of the middle zone of the medial meniscus. 109: Wedge shaped stump after oblique tear of the posterior horn (interrupted line = bursa semimembranosogastrocne mica. 110: Small irregular defect on the undersurface of the meniscus.

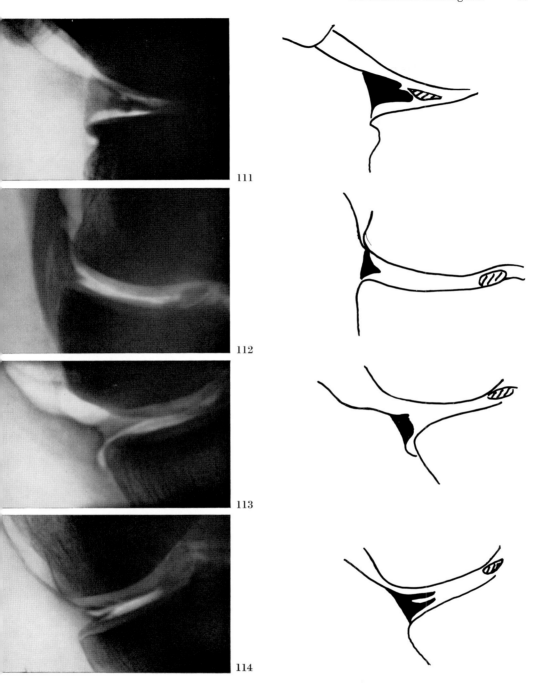

Figs. 111–114. *Meniscus defects*. Torn fragments visible in the interior of the joint (crosshatched). Meniscus stump (black). 111: Anterior horn, medial meniscus, minimal displacement of the fragment. 112: Middle zone, medial meniscus. Stump very small and wedge-shaped, marked displacement of the fragment. 113: Flattened stump imbibed with contrast medium (old bucket handle tear). 114: A detached fragment from the inner border of the meniscus. Fork-shaped stump.

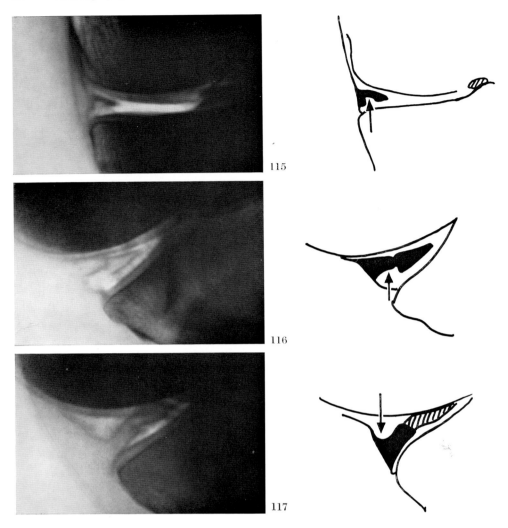

Figs. 115–117. *Meniscus defects* (arrows point to the defects). 115: Defect on the undersurface of the medial meniscus, middle zone. The torn fragment is visible in the interior of the joint (crosshatched). 116: Defects in the undersurface of the posterior horn of the medial meniscus close to the capsule. 117: Defect in the upper surface of the meniscus close to the capsule. Fragment (crosshatched) displaced into the interior of the joint. Typical junction between bucket and handle in the posterior horn of the medial meniscus.

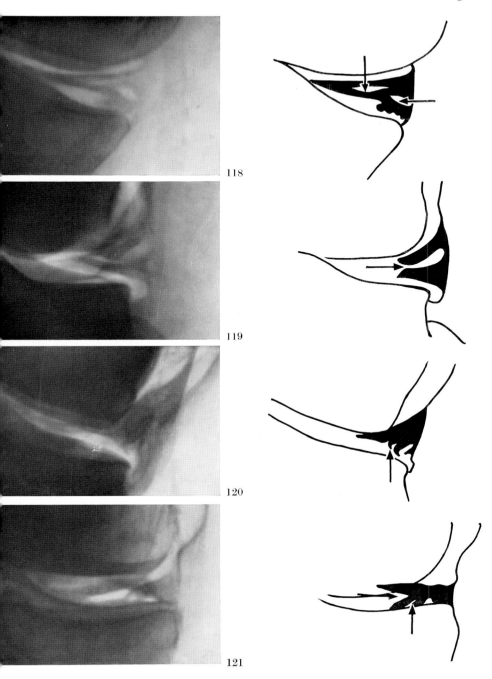

Figs. 118–121. *Fragmentation of the meniscus* (lateral): 118: Tear formation within the meniscus. 119: Horizontal split. 120: Vertical fragmentation of the undersurface. 121: Fragmentation and separation of the fragments.

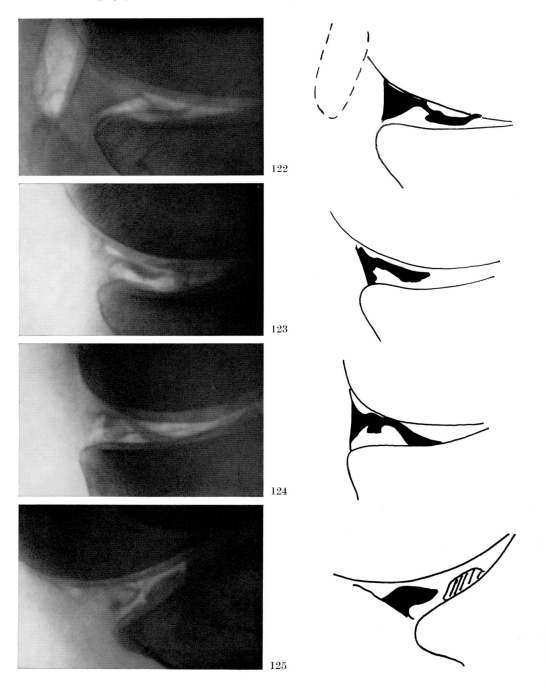

Figs. 122–125. *Destruction and fragmentation of the meniscus*. 122–124: Formation of tongue-shaped fragments in the posterior horn of the medial meniscus. 125: Destruction and detachment. Free fragments crosshatched.

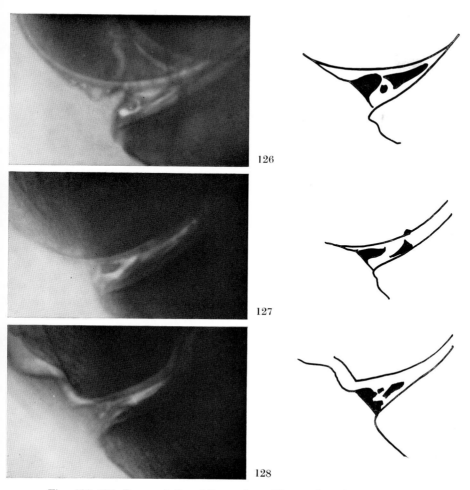

126

127

128

Figs. 126–128. *Fragmentation of the meniscus.* The meniscus is torn into several fragments.

or degenerative changes of the fragments such as a ragged appearance and imbibition (Figs. 79, 121).

*Indirect signs*

Arthritic osteophyte formations on the bone adjacent to an old injury can be seen on the routine X-ray view. The cartilage surrounding the lesion is thinned out (Fig. 79).

## 2) Degenerative Meniscus Changes

The arthrogram of the meniscus can show symptoms which can be interpreted as signs of degenerative changes (Schnauder):

*a) Imbibition* of the edges with liquid contrast medium (Fig. 129). The liquid contrast medium permeates the inferior and superior surface of the meniscus because the covering epithelium is destroyed and the tissue underneath it is necrotic and fragmented.

*b) Fragmentation* (Fig. 130). This is usually found on the undersurface of the meniscus and may be due to degenerative changes in the cartilaginous surface of the tibial plateau.

*c) Flattening of the meniscus* (Figs. 131–132). The meniscus is flattened out to a thin plate in its cranio-caudal diameter or its surface is rolled out in a concave manner. The contours are sharply delineated and smooth. These changes

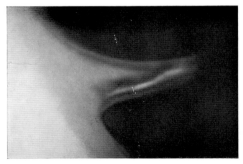 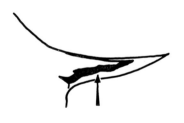

Fig. 129. Degeneration of the meniscus, posterior horn of the medial meniscus. Imbibition with liquid contrast medium on the undersurface of the meniscus produces thickening and blurriness of the contours (arrow).

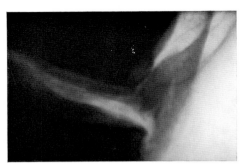 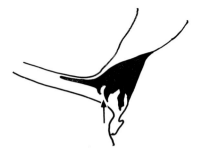

Fig. 130. Degenerated meniscus. Middle zone of the lateral meniscus with fragmentation of the undersurface (arrow).

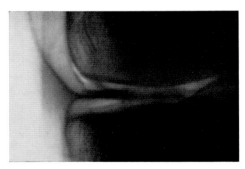 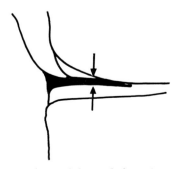

Fig. 131. Degenerated and flattened meniscus (anterior horn of the medial meniscus).

can be seen especially on those fragments which are constantly subjected to the grinding motions between femur and tibia.

*d) Thickening* of the meniscus (Figs. 133, 134). The cross section of the meniscus resembles a bottle whose neck is directed towards the interior of the joint. These changes are usually caused by cyst formation.

*e) Meniscus ganglion.* This represents a cystic degeneration of the cartilaginous tissue (Fig. 135).

It is frequently combined with a horizontal tear of the meniscus (Lindblom). The cross section of the meniscus is rather high and occasionally has convex contours. The body of the meniscus frequently contains cysts which are connected with the joint by a tear or a slot. The arthrogram of a cyst with a tear resembles a tennis racquet (Ficat).

Degenerative meniscus changes are frequently associated with arthritic cartilage or bone

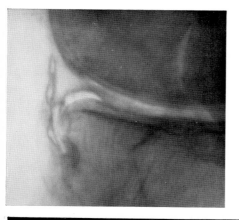

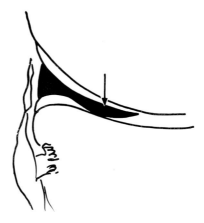

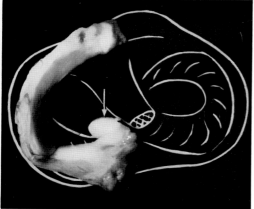

Fig. 132. Partially detached posterior horn fragment flattened in a typical manner. Above: Arthrogram: Thinning of the posterior horn of the medial meniscus, continues into the flattened portion (arrow) which is concave on the cranial and convex on the caudal surface. This corresponds to the small flattened fragment of the surgical specimen below (arrow).

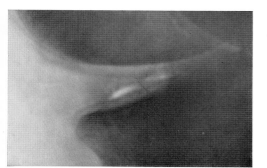

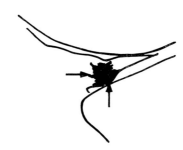

Fig. 133. Degeneration (medial meniscus, posterior horn). Enlargement of the meniscus (vertical arrow) and imbibition with contrast medium (horizontal arrow). Histology: Mucoid degeneration.

lesions. Both lesions probably have a tendency to aggravate each other. Marked degenerative bone and cartilage changes in the vicinity of a meniscus lesion have been demonstrated by Jonasch and Lindblom. Calcifications of the meniscus (Fig. 136) are degenerative changes and can frequently be seen on routine x-rays in conjunction with arthritic changes.

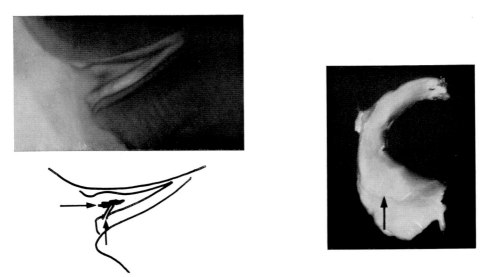

Fig. 134. Degeneration of the posterior horn of the medial meniscus. Left: Arthrogram: Imbibition (horizontal arrow) and slight swelling with tear (vertical arrow) in the same area (undersurface). This is probably a tear following primary degeneration in a 54-year-old housewife without any history of injury. Right: A small tear is visible next to the surface of the surgical specimen (arrow).

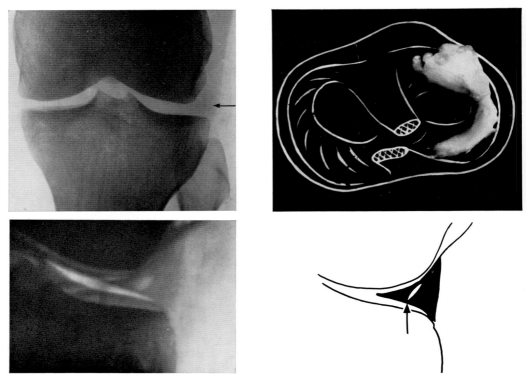

Fig. 135. Meniscus ganglion at the junction between the anterior horn and the middle zone of the lateral meniscus. This can be visualized quite well on the regular X-ray: The lateral joint space is slightly widened. There is a circumscribed soft tissue swelling adjacent to the joint space (arrow). Below left: Arthrogram: Marked enlargement of the meniscus wedge with oval-shaped radiolucency in the center (arrow). Right: Surgical specimen. Marked enlargement of the anterior horn.

### 3) Developmental Anomalies of the Menisci

The mesenchymal junction between femur and tibia in the embryo gradually develops into two primitive joint spaces, one on the femoral side and one on the tibial side. They are separated by a horizontal septum whose peripheral portions later develop into the menisci (Hamilton et al.). The central portions regress. The extent of this regression determines the shape of the meniscus, and can produce a complete or incomplete discoid meniscus, a deformed or a hypoplastic meniscus (Fig. 137).

Abnormal menisci may produce vague complaints in the knee. They can form the basis for the development of a meniscus ganglion and are very prone to injuries (Jeannopoulos, Rieunau and Ficat, Smillie, Catolla). Developmental anomalies of the meniscus are more frequent on the lateral than on the medial side. The *arthrogram* of a complete discoid meniscus (Fig. 137a) has a band-like appearance instead of the wedge-shaped cross section of the normal meniscus. It occupies the entire half of the joint and separates the femoral and tibial condyles completely (Fig. 138).

A *ring-shaped* meniscus (Fig. 137b, c) also represents a developmental anomaly. It can be distinguished in the arthrogram from a bucket-handle tear by the normal appearance of its outer portion unless there are additional injuries (Fig. 139).

The *infantile discoid* meniscus (Smillie) (Fig. 137d) has an anterior and posterior horn of normal size. Its middle zone, however, extends far into the interior of the joint and can be demonstrated quite well in the arthrogram (Fig. 140).

The arthrogram of a *partial discoid* meniscus (Fig. 137e) shows a wider than normal cross section extending farther into the interior of the joint (Fig. 141).

Occasionally there can be *excessive enlargement of the posterior horn* of the meniscus (Fig. 137f) for which Ficat has coined the term *"ménisque en virgule inversée"*.

Middleton mentions another developmental deformity – a *comma-shaped meniscus* with an enlarged anterior horn. The *hypoplastic or small*

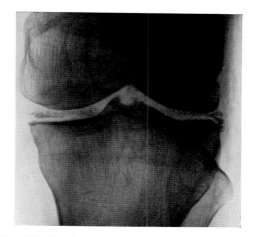

Fig. 136. Calcification of the meniscus, regular X-ray.

*meniscus* shows a remarkably small wedge-shaped shadow, especially in its anterior horn and middle portions, which resembles a meniscus remnant or a regenerated meniscus after meniscectomy.

Meniscus anomalies often come to our attention after the patient has sustained an injury to his knee. Horizontal tears (Fig. 140) are frequent and are occasionally combined with a ganglion. These patients usually show some arthritic changes despite their relatively young age.

## F. Status Post-Meniscectomy

Surgical meniscectomy usually does not remove the meniscus totally but leaves a small well-vascularized pericapsular zone, the so-called zone of regeneration. A meniscus-like structure with a wedge-shaped cross section regenerates from this zone shortly after the operation. This wedge is smaller and shorter with a broad base towards the capsule and usually has sharp contours (Figs. 142–147). The wedge can be slightly asymmetric with its upper leg shorter or longer than the lower (Fig. 145). Its inner edge is frequently blunt.

Even after total meniscectomy the arthrogram rarely shows a straight vertical capsular wall. Most of the time a small short meniscus wedge remains which, however, in the arthrogram and

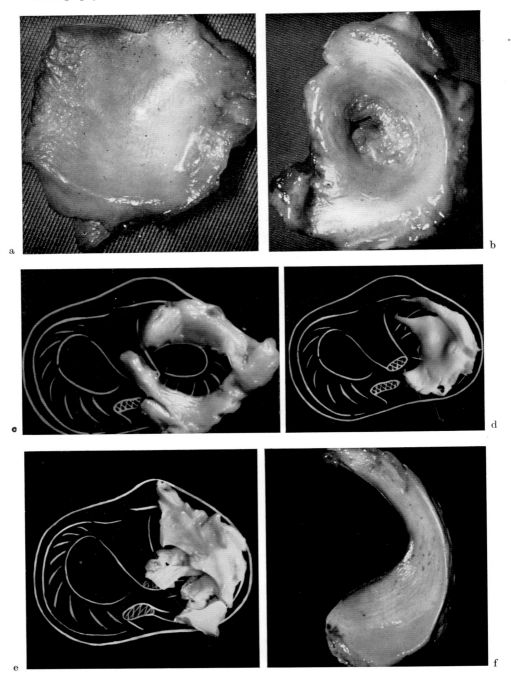

Fig. 137. *Developmental anomalies of the meniscus* (surgical specimens). a) Discoid meniscus. b) Ring-shaped meniscus (some central resorption). c) Ring-shaped meniscus (marked central resorption) with tear in the inner portion. d) So-called infantile meniscus (Smillie): central portion not resorbed. e) Crescent-shaped meniscus, torn. f) Comma-shaped meniscus (enlarged posterior horn). A comma-shaped meniscus with large anterior horn (Middleton) is not available in our material. (a, b, d, from Catolla).

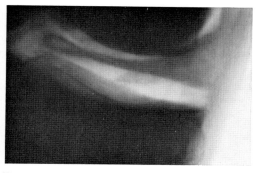
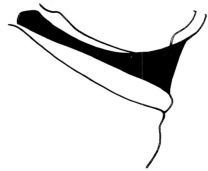

Fig. 138. Complete discoid meniscus, arthrogram. Band-shaped shadow (black), which is thinner in the center, extends from the capsule to the middle of the joint (see Fig. 137 a).

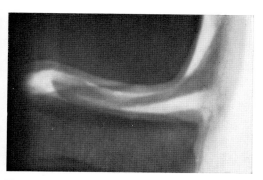
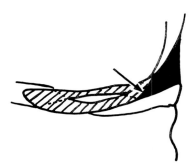

Fig. 139. Ring-shaped meniscus. The open center is faintly visible in the arthrogram (arrow). The outer ring portion has a sharp inner corner (black). The inner portions of the ring are crosshatched (see Fig. 137 b, c).

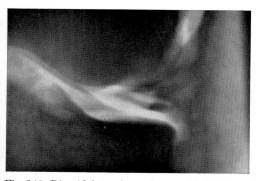
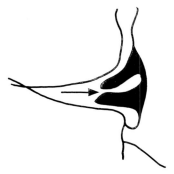

Fig. 140. Discoid lateral meniscus with horizontal tear (arrow) (corresponds to Fig. 98). (See Fig. 137 d.)

even at operation resembles more a capsular fold than a meniscus remnant (Fig. 146).

After partial meniscectomy the regenerated meniscus is usually wider (Figs. 147–151). Its cross section is usually wedge-shaped and sometimes plump, especially in the posterior horn region (Fig. 153).

After a difficult and uneven resection of the meniscus the remnant may occasionally produce a bizarre shadow (Figs. 150–153).

Arthrography makes a good postoperative evaluation of the type of meniscectomy possible and can reveal inadequacies of the performed operation. We know from experience that it is

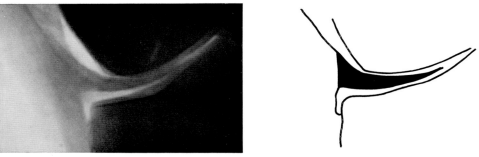

Fig. 141. Crescent-shaped meniscus. The meniscus wedge (black) extends from the capsule to the middle of the articular surface (see Fig. 137e).

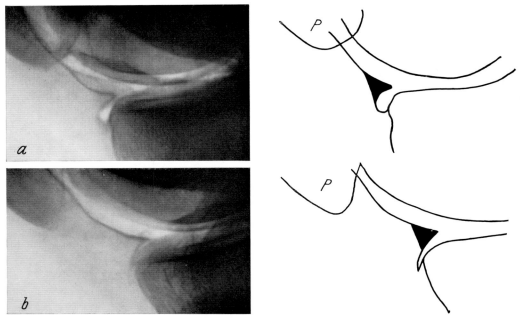

Fig. 142. Anterior horn remnant after medial meniscectomy. a) Surgery 3 years ago, short wedge-shaped shadow, dull inner border, sharp contours. b) Surgery 4½ years ago, pointed inner border.

impossible to visualize the posterior horn from a small anterior incision and believe that for evaluation of the posterior horn, arthrography is superior to surgical exploration. The posterior horn should be left in the joint only when it is intact (Rutscheidt); however, frequently the posterior horn is involved in the lesion. Complaints after meniscectomy which persist or increase should not be put aside as inevitable postmeniscectomy complaints. Quite often they are due to an incompletely removed torn posterior horn. We have a good number of examples in our own material (Figs. 154–158).

## G. Sources of Diagnostic Errors

Errors in the examination and in the X-ray technic, as well as erroneous interpretation of anatomic details in the arthrogram, are frequent

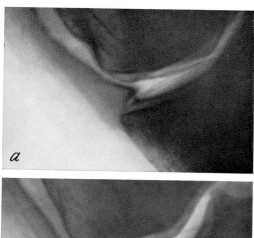

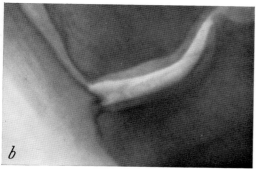

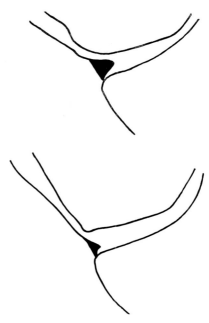

Fig. 143. Status post medial meniscectomy, middle zone. a) Surgery 3 years ago, shortened pointed wedge, sharp contours. b) Surgery 8 years ago, small asymmetric, dull wedge.

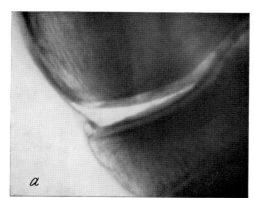

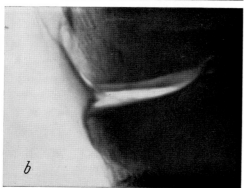

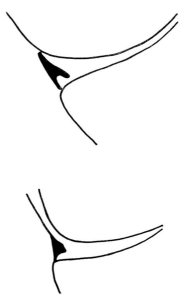

Fig. 144. Status after so-called total meniscectomy. Middle zone. a) Surgery 6 months ago, small asymmetric wedge. b) Surgery 3 years ago, very short, dull wedge, resembling a capsular fold.

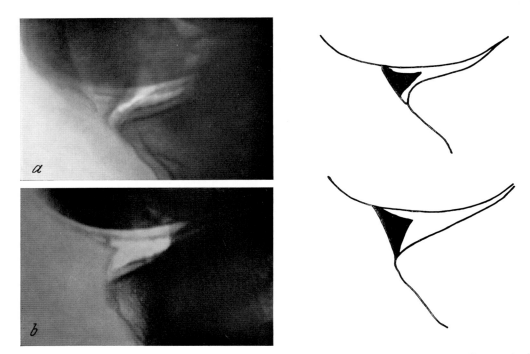

Fig. 145. Status after medial meniscectomy, posterior horn. a) Surgery 6 months ago, small posterior horn remnant, short and sharply delineated. b) Surgery 3 years ago, asymmetric, short wedge.

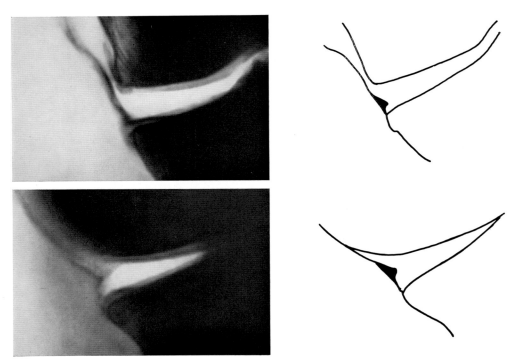

Fig. 146. Status after so-called total medial meniscectomy 7 months ago. a) Anterior horn, asymmetric flat wedge, which looks more like a capsular fold than a meniscus remnant. b) Posterior horn: flat wedge resembling a capsular fold.

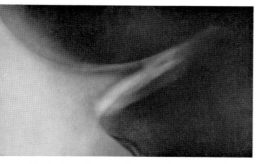
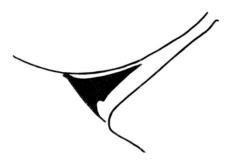

Fig. 147. Status after medial meniscectomy. Incomplete removal of the posterior horn. Relatively large posterior horn remnant, pointed, wedge-shaped shadow. Infra-meniscal space widened.

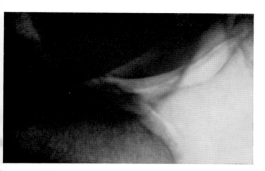
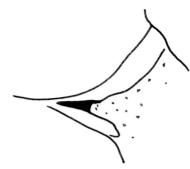

Fig. 148. Status post lateral meniscectomy, 4½ years ago. The anterior horn can be recognized as a short wedge with a pointed inner border (black). (Regenerated meniscus?)

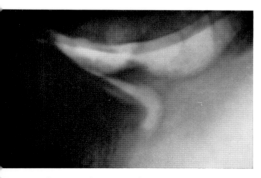
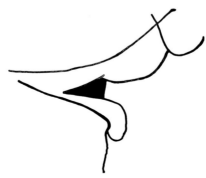

Fig. 149. Status after lateral meniscectomy approximately 3½ years ago. The anterior horn is visible as a relatively large wedge. It must be assumed that the meniscus was only partially removed; the arthrographic findings resemble those of a normal lateral anterior horn (see Fig. 40).

causes of false diagnoses. In the following chapter the pitfalls of arthrographic diagnoses will be discussed briefly. These chapters are based on experience gained from our own mistakes and from working with trainees who were learning the double contrast method. It is obvious that the method has its limitations and even an experienced examiner can make mistakes. We are of the opinion, however, that most of these mistakes can be avoided by strict observation of the points discussed in this chapter.

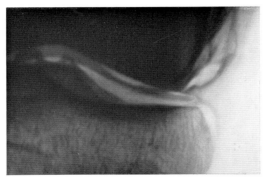
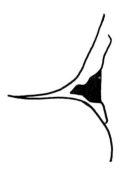

Fig. 150. Status post lateral meniscectomy, 4 ½ years ago. Middle zone. The meniscus remnant has a tongue-shaped appearance.

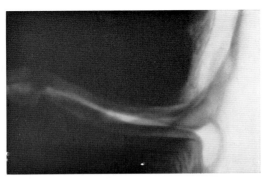
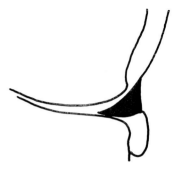

Fig. 151. Status post lateral meniscectomy 3 years ago. Middle zone. Relatively broad, wedge-shaped shadow. (Meniscus remnant or regenerated meniscus?)

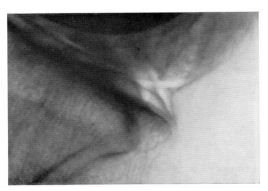
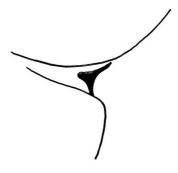

Fig. 152. Status post lateral meniscectomy 4 ½ years ago. Posterior horn (black), short asymmetric wedge.

## 1) Errors in Technic

### a) Periarticular Injection of Contrast Medium

Periarticular injections of liquid contrast medium are usually made into the fatty tissue between the suprapatellar pouch and the anterior surface of the femur (see Fig. 37). This results in a pure air arthrogram and poor delineation of the interior structures of the knee. The error is easily detected under fluoroscopy. A

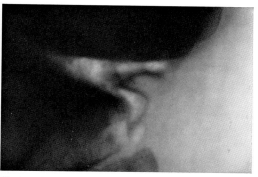 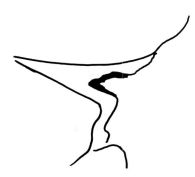

Fig. 153. Status post lateral meniscectomy. The plump posterior horn remnant is stained with contrast medium.

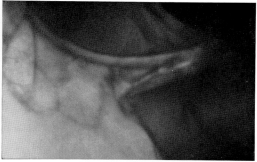

Fig. 154. Status post meniscectomy. Above: Arthrogram. Posterior horn remnant which has torn loose from its capsular attachment (crosshatched). Right: Surgical specimen. The posterior horn remnant is detached from the capsule in its entire length; the torn border of the meniscus is smooth.

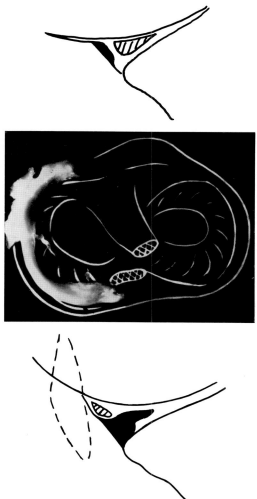

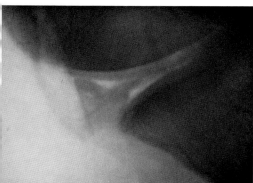

Fig. 155. Status post medial meniscectomy 9 years ago. Posterior horn remnant (black). A torn fragment (crosshatched) is visible in the superior capsular space. Interrupted line: bursa semimembranosogastrocnemica.

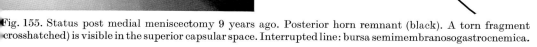

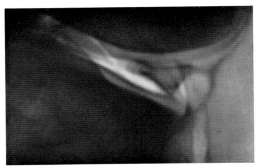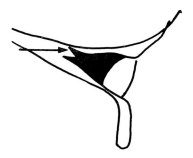

Fig. 156. Status post lateral meniscectomy 6 years ago. Posterior horn remnant with small horizontal tear of its inner border (arrow).

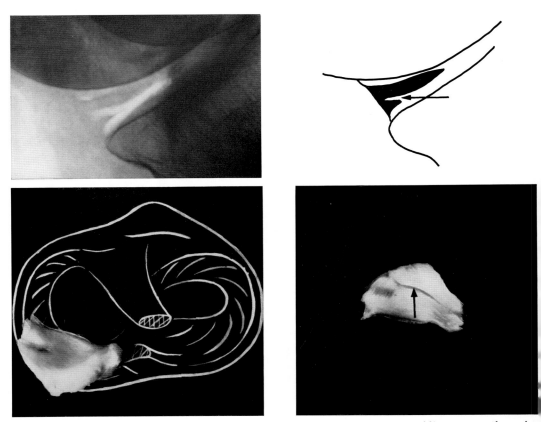

Fig. 157. Status post medial meniscectomy 9 years ago. Posterior horn remnant with oblique tear on the under-surface. Above: Arthrogram: The arrow points to the tear. Below: Surgical specimen. Left: Superior surface of the meniscus remnant. Right: Undersurface of the meniscus remnant; the tear is clearly visible (arrow).

second correctly placed injection of contrast medium remedies the situation. Periarticular injection of liquid contrast medium into the area of the collateral ligaments could lead to a false diagnosis of a ligamentous tear. Periarticular injection of air produces an emphysema of the soft tissues. Excessive injection of air has the same effect. Rapidly developing tears in the serosa will allow the air to penetrate into the surrounding tissues (see Fig. 38). The air can

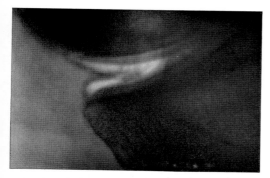

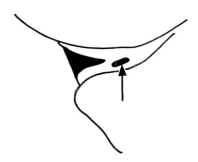

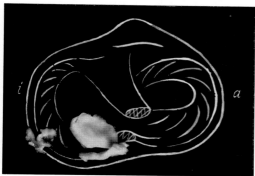

Fig. 158. Status post medial meniscectomy 3 years ago. Posterior horn remnant with small detached fragment. Above: Arthrogram, fragment (arrow). Below: Surgical specimen, meniscus remnant posteriorly with the small fragment adjacent to it.

permeate into the pericapsular or perimeniscal regions and cause disturbing superimpositions which can be confused with ligamentous lesions. The areas of periarticular air injection can be recognized, however, because they contain only air and no liquid contrast medium. Their location does not always coincide with that of the capsule as in a true ligamentous lesion (Fig. 159).

### b) Incomplete Evacuation of Joint Effusions

Excess joint fluid will dilute the contrast medium. This results in blurring of the contours, and small tears can be overlooked (Fig. 160). The examination should be repeated and the liquid contrast medium should not be injected until the joint effusion has been evacuated completely (see Fig. 28).

### 2) Errors in X-ray Technic

#### a) Projection Not Orthograde

The use of the fluoroscope facilitates orthograde projection of the meniscus. The meniscotibial space can then be visualized as a clear, air-containing band. When the tube is focused poorly, the central ray will not penetrate the meniscus at its cross section but rather slightly obliquely from a cranial or caudal direction. This causes disturbing superimposition (Figs. 161–162) which can easily be confused with a meniscus lesion. Only orthograde projections of the meniscus should be used for diagnostic purposes.

#### b) Excessive Rotation

Excessive external rotation to visualize the posterior horn of the medial meniscus may cause a superimposition of the posterior horn of the lateral meniscus over that of the medial meniscus. Projection of the hiatus popliteus of the posterior horn of the lateral meniscus into the medial meniscus could cause misinterpretation (Fig. 163).

These overlapping effects always show the same appearance and location of the tibial and femoral condyles helps to recognize this error.

### 3) Errors in the Anatomical Differentiation of the Arthrogram

#### a) Superimposition of the Infrapatellar Fat Pad

The infrapatellar fat pad reaches into the joint space in a tongue-shaped fashion caudally. This

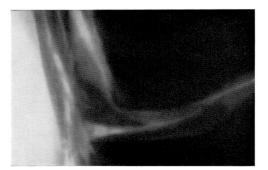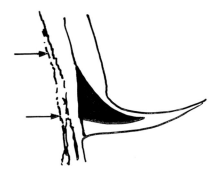

Fig. 159. Periarticular air infiltration. Broad parameniscal air shadows (arrows), no leakage of contrast medium (lateral view, see Fig. 38).

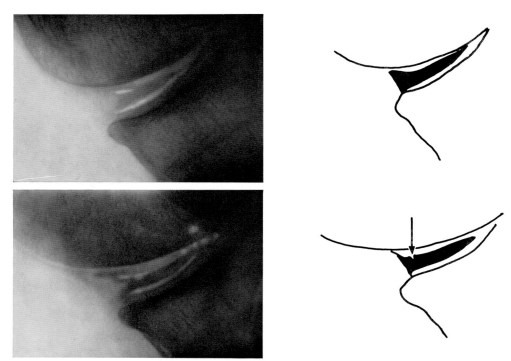

Fig. 160. Above: Joint effusion not evacuated completely resulting in blurry contours of the meniscus with poor contrast. Below: Arthrogram after complete evacuation of the joint effusion. The contrast is much better, the meniscus is delineated more sharply, a small tear on the upper surface is now visible (arrow).

caudal tongue can have varying shapes (Figs. 69–71) and can occasionally resemble the cross section of a meniscus but with a rounded off inner border. The tongue-shaped portion of the infrapatellar fat pad can occasionally overlie the anterior horn of the medial meniscus in such a fashion as to simulate a tear (see Fig. 167). Occasionally the fat pad may have villi which can,

by superimposition, simulate lesions of the anterior horn of the medial meniscus (Fig. 164).

b) Superimposition of the Recessus

The recessus are usually evenly shaped, well rounded indentations of the menisci near their capsular attachment and should not be confused

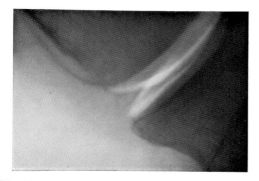
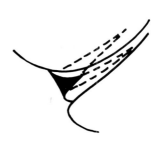

Fig. 161. Meniscus not in orthograde projection, middle zone medial meniscus. The wedge-shaped shadow (black) is clearly visible and appears intact. The overlying portions of the meniscus (interrupted line) do not represent a pathologic finding.

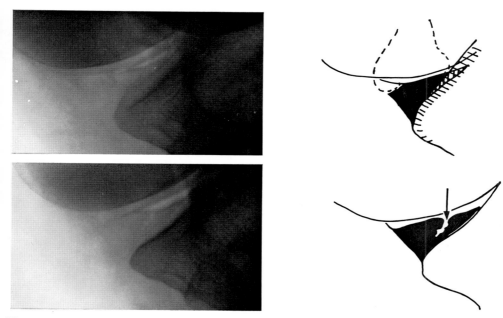

Fig. 162. Above: Posterior horn of medial meniscus not in orthograde projection. The meniscus is partially obscured by the tibial plateau (crossed area) and cannot be evaluated properly. Interrupted line: Bursa. Below: The same meniscus as above in a better projection. A tear is now clearly visible (arrow).

with tears. Occasionally we observe more extensive recessus formations which could be diagnosed erroneously as marginal tears of the meniscus (Fig. 165). The significance of these large recessus is not yet fully understood. One could postulate that these formations represent old tears which are partially scarred as pointed out by Schaer. One could also postulate that these large recessus represent excessive mobility of the meniscus

*(laxité du ménisque, ménisque allongé)*. We suggest a classification of these recessus into well rounded, smoothly shaped anatomic recessus and suspicious pathologic forms (large, perhaps unevenly shaped recessi). Occasionally we find the entrance to a bursa situated in one of these recessus which may resemble a tear in the meniscus (see Figs. 67, 68).

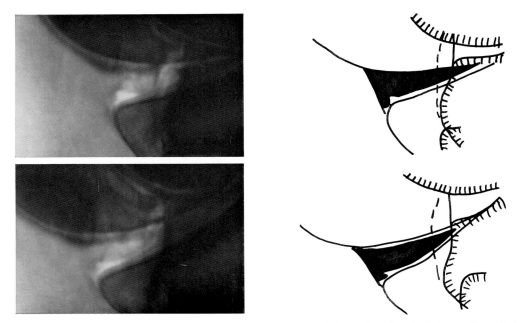

Fig. 163. Excessive rotation. Above: This is almost a lateral view. The tendon sheath of the popliteus (interrupted line) of the lateral meniscus is superimposed on the inner border of the medial meniscus. The contours of the lateral tibial condyle and the lateral femoral condyle and also those of the head of the fibula are crosshatched (see Fig. 63).

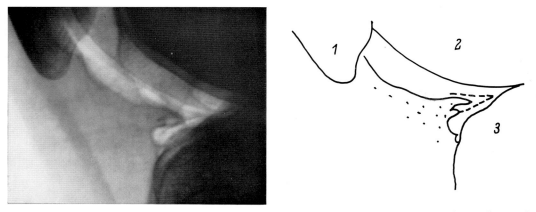

Fig. 164. Superimposition of Hoffa's fat pad. The villous Hoffa's fat pad (dotted) is superimposed over the anterior horn of the medial meniscus (interrupted line). The meniscus is intact.

### c) Superimposition of a Bursa

Superimposition of a bursa is usually not disturbing since the bursa is not filled with liquid contrast medium and is visualized as an air-containing, sharply contoured space (see Fig. 47).

We have already mentioned that the entrance to a bursa can permeate a meniscus near its capsular attachment. It shows smooth and even contours with the shadow of the adjoining bursa attached to it and should not be confused with a tear (see Fig. 68).

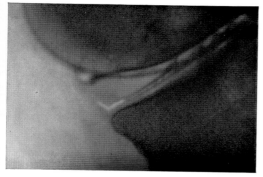

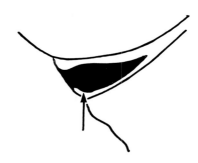

Fig. 165. Recessus. A very deep, smoothly delineated and slightly rounded recessus (arrow) is seen at the junction of the undersurface of the meniscus and the capsule. This is not a pathologic finding, but may result in excessive mobility and increased vulnerability of the meniscus. A small, shallow recessus is present at the junction between the capsule and the superior surface of the meniscus.

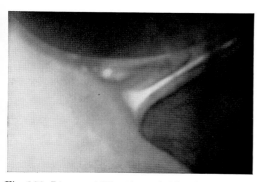

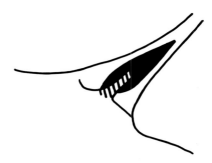

Fig. 166. Ligament-like tissue bridge between capsule and posterior horn of the meniscus (see Fig. 48). Anatomic finding.

### d) Connection of the Posterior Horn of the Medial Meniscus with the Capsule

This small ligament (Rüttimann) has a very typical appearance and should not be confused with a tear (see Fig. 166). Its presence usually means some relaxation and increased mobility of the posterior horn.

### e) The Popliteal Hiatus

The anatomical configuration of this hiatus varies very little (see Figs. 54 and 55) and it is very rarely confused with a tear. Excessive rotation can occasionally superimpose it over the medial meniscus and lead to the false diagnosis of a meniscus tear (see Fig. 163).

### f) Our Own Errors

Our own series shows a 5 per cent incidence of diagnostic errors (28 false diagnoses in 625 operative cases). Catolla reported an error rate of only 3 per cent with the same method. We were present at operation in approximately one-half of these cases. The remaining 50 per cent were verified by the operative report of the surgeon and the histologic examination. In most cases the missed or falsely diagnosed lesion could be detected in the arthrogram retrospectively. Most of these diagnostic errors were made by us and our co-workers in the beginning. They were usually due to avoidable causes such as technically inadequate arthrograms and false anatomical interpretation. The number of cases where the lesion could not be detected in the arthrogram is very small (transverse meniscus tears!). Figures 167–174 demonstrate some of our misinterpretations.

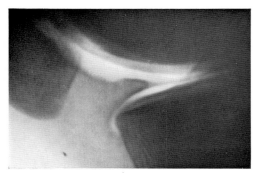 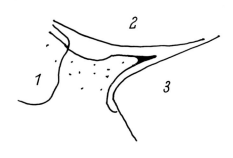

Fig. 167. False diagnosis: Hoffa's fat pad (dotted) was diagnosed as a pathologically shortened anterior horn of the medial meniscus. The normal pointed inner border of the meniscus (black) was overlooked. 1. Patella. 2. Femur. 3. Tibia.

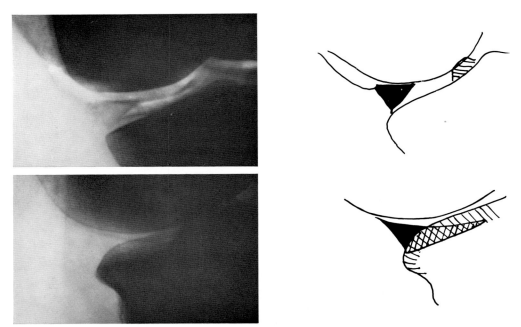

Fig. 168. False diagnosis: Medial meniscus. Above: Pathology in the anterior horn (black) cannot be visualized with certainty. The fragment (crosshatched) in the interior of the joint should not have been overlooked. Below: Posterior horn, not in orthograde projection. Only a portion is clearly visualized (black); the remaining portion (crossed) is obscured by the head of the tibia and cannot be evaluated. The posterior horn was torn.

## H. Complications of Double Contrast Arthrography

We have not seen any serious complications in a series of approximately 2500 arthrographies.

Occasionally we see a joint effusion, especially in patients who have had recurring joint effusions before the arthrogram. These effusions are present for several days and disappear spontaneously. Pain is rare. We have seen painful muscle emphysema due to excessive injection of air into the joint in two patients. The complaints disappeared within two days. One patient developed edema of the ankle after arthrography (angioneurotic?) which disappeared overnight with elevation of the leg.

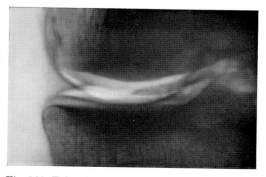
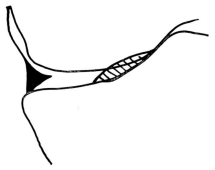

Fig. 169. False diagnosis: Middle zone, medial meniscus. The meniscus wedge (black) appears very small, but could be within normal limits. The torn fragment (crosshatched) in the interior of the joint was overlooked.

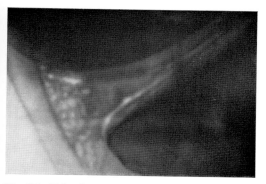
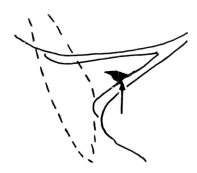

Fig. 170. False diagnosis: Medial meniscus, posterior horn. The bursa semimembranosogastrocnemica (crosshatched) contains air bubbles. The small tear on the undersurface of the meniscus (arrow) in a degenerated zone (imbibed with contrast medium) was overlooked.

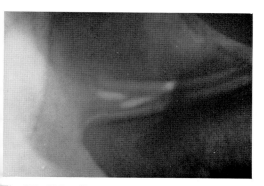
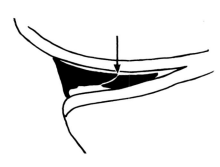

Fig. 171. False diagnosis: Medial meniscus, posterior horn. The oblique tear (arrow) was overlooked because of poor contrast effect (see Fig. 160).

Allergic reactions can occur with injection of any contrast medium. We have seen this in one patient who developed urticaria of the entire body and asthma-like complaints which disappeared within two days after treatment with calcium and antihistamines. No significant complications should be expected if all precautions discussed in the chapter on methodology are observed.

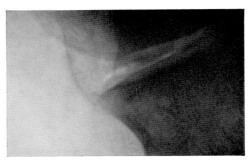 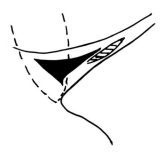

Fig. 172. False diagnosis: Medial meniscus, posterior horn. Bursa semimembranosogastrocnemica (interrupted line). The free fragment (crosshatched) was overlooked. Poor contrast effect because of inadequade evacuation of the effusion.

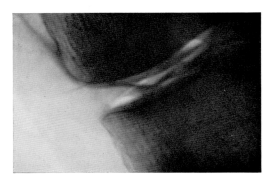 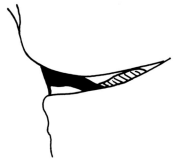

Fig. 173. False diagnosis: Medial meniscus, middle zone. The torn fragment (crosshatched) in the interior of the joint was overlooked. The atypical form of the meniscus stump (black) should have made the examiner suspicious.

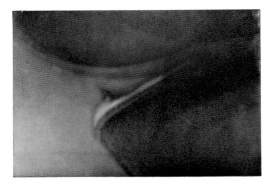 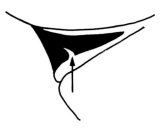

Fig. 174. A tear on the undersurface was diagnosed by the radiologist. The operating surgeon, however, did not agree with this finding. Histologic examination confirmed the finding of an old tear. Excision of the meniscus had been carried out through the tear.

# I. Radiation Exposure

## 1) Exposure of the Patient

Lars-Eric Larson conducted extensive examinations to determine radiation exposure of the patient during arthrography of the knee joint. The settings used by him, the number of exposures and the film focus distance of 70 cm. are approximately the same as ours. The film focus distance in our series varied up to 90 cm. and our pictures are of smaller size. These small differences should not significantly alter the testicular dose of 6.5 mr. and the ovarial dose of 1 to 2 mr. as given by Larson. These measurements show that the risk of gonadal damage from arthrography is minimal for the patient and that the procedure is justified.

## 2) Radiation Exposure of the Examiner

We have measured the radiation exposure of the examiner with film dosimetry. This examination has shown that radiation exposure of the examiner is very minimal as long as he is correctly protected with lead gloves and a lead apron. Care must be taken, however, that the examiner's hands are not exposed to the main X-ray beam which can occur when the knee is passively rotated or the fluoroscopy screen is moved.

CHAPTER 6

# Clinical and Radiologic Differential Diagnosis

This chapter is a discussion of differential diagnostic considerations when a meniscus lesion is suspected. Schaer has pointed out that traumatic locking or characteristic recurrences rarely give rise to diagnostic difficulties. Chronic irritations of the knee joint with constant but changing complaints, intermittent hydrops and unclear clinical findings are much more difficult to diagnose but are frequently due to a meniscus lesion. Experience has shown that physicians tend to make a diagnosis of meniscus lesions too often rather than not often enough. A typical meniscus lesion very rarely simulates another condition but there are a number of other afflictions of the knee joint with unclear symptoms which could be confused with a meniscus lesion, especially in their beginning stages.

It is mandatory, therefore, to consider all differential diagnostic possibilities before we open a joint for surgical intervention. There are a number of joint conditions which can be influenced unfavorably by a poorly indicated arthrotomy. An unstable knee for instance, can sometimes be made more unstable by operative intervention because the quadriceps atrophy which follows the operation tends to increase instability. Arthrosis of the knee joint can be made more painful by an operation.

Some of the conditions listed here can usually be differentiated from a meniscus lesion without difficulty with the help of the history and clinical examination. Arthrography often gives us valuable additional information.

## 1) Ligamentous and Capsular Damage

### a) Collateral Ligament and Capsule Lesions

Ligaments, joint capsule and menisci form a functional unit. Injuries to the knee joint frequently produce combined lesions of collateral and cruciate ligaments, the capsule and the menisci which are difficult to differentiate, especially in the early stages.

Usually the symptoms and signs of collateral ligament lesions predominate in these cases. Si-

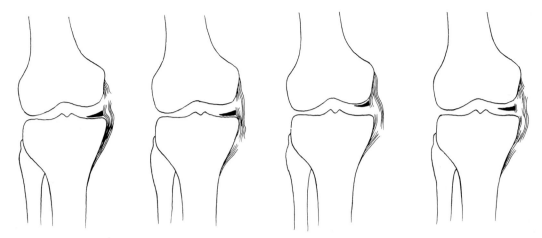

Fig. 175. Different forms of collateral ligament lesions (modified from Smillie).

milar to traumatic lesions of the menisci, injuries to the collateral ligaments occur from indirect trauma with forced rotation in slight flexion. This can occur when the body is rotated forcefully on the fixed foot or when the foot suddenly slips out from under the body. We observe these torsion injuries most frequently in skiers. Forced adduction or abduction of the leg in full extension can also injure the collateral ligament. This can occur in a soccer game when a player falls over the outstretched leg of another player. Because of the physiologic valgus position of the knee joint, the medial collateral ligament is more vulnerable than the less tense lateral collateral ligament.

The *clinical picture* of a collateral ligament injury depends on the severity of the lesion. Simple *sprains* which stretch but do not tear the ligament, need not produce any swelling or effusion. In contrast to a meniscus lesion, mobility of the knee is frequently not limited in the first few hours after the injury and some weight can be borne on the knee joint. We always find circumscribed tenderness over the collateral ligament. On the medial side, this tenderness is usually located above the joint space over the femoral attachment of the ligament. Stability of the joint is not impaired as long as the ligamentous injury is not severe. The joint space cannot be opened. The attempted distraction of the joint space, however, is painful because of the pull on the injured ligament. Compression of the joint space would produce pain if a meniscus lesion were present (Böhler's sign).

A partial or total *tear* of the medial collateral ligament will automatically produce an injury of the joint capsule (Fig. 175). This usually leads to an extra-articular hematoma and a joint effusion which can develop very rapidly when a severe ligamentous and capsular injury is present. The lateral collateral ligament is not connected with the joint capsule and capsular injuries are less frequent on the lateral side. When a complete tear of the collateral ligament is present, the joint can be opened without pain. Severe distortions of the knee with extensive injuries to ligaments and capsule produce a more diffuse tenderness with increased tenderness over the joint line when the middle section of the ligament is injured (Fig. 175).

After injury to the collateral ligament, the knee joint is often held in a position of slight flexion to relax the injured ligamentous and capsular structures. Poor positioning of the joint will lead rapidly to contracture of the capsule and to a limitation extension, which is difficult to distinguish from true locking after a meniscus lesion. A ligamentous injury, however, will also cause limitation of flexion in most cases.

An old inadequately treated ligamentous injury produces instability of the knee joint. Similar to meniscus tears these patients complain of

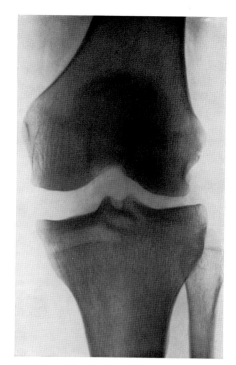

Fig. 176. Stress film. Lesion of the collateral ligament. Diastasis of the medial joint space.

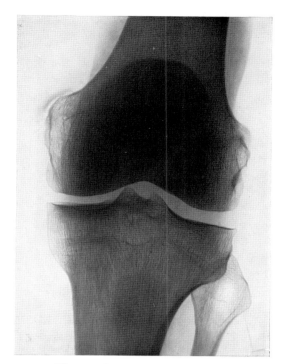

Fig. 177. Pellegrini-Stieda shadow.

sudden "giving way" episodes when they walk downstairs or down a slope with uncontrolled motions, etc.

This frequently makes it very difficult to distinguish meniscus and ligamentous injuries and may make it impossible in a fresh injury to determine whether a meniscus lesion exists in addition to a ligamentous injury.

The previously described Apley test sometimes helps in the differential diagnosis. Occasionally it is of benefit to anesthetize the point of tenderness over the collateral ligament attachment by extra-articular injection of a local anesthetic. If a previously existing limitation of extension disappears after this local anesthesia and no meniscus signs are present, the possibility of internal derangement of the knee is rather remote.

In each severe injury to the knee the clinical examination should be supplemented by routine X-ray examination. Occasionally fresh injuries of the collateral ligaments can be detected by visualization of small cortical avulsion fractures from the epicondyles of the femur or the head

of the fibula. Stress films in abduction and adduction reveal abnormal widening of the joint space when the collateral ligament is partially or completely torn (Fig. 176).

The so-called *Pellegrini-Stieda-shadow* is a sure sign of an old collateral ligament lesion. The shadow represents soft tissue calcification adjacent to the femoral condyle (Fig. 177). It is irregular or sickle-shaped and cannot be detected by X-ray until 2 weeks after the injury. Its size and structure can change in the first few months. Typical signs of a ligamentous tear on the *arthrogram* are: 1) formation of tears or slots in the capsule; 2) widening of the menisco-tibial and/or meniscofemoral joint space with the appropriate passive knee motion (adduction or abduction) (Figs. 180, 181).

The medial collateral ligament is firmly attached to the joint capsule; the lateral is not. A tear of the medial collateral ligament always produces a tear of the capsule. Collateral ligament or capsular tears are visualized in the arthrogram as spaces which are filled with positive contrast

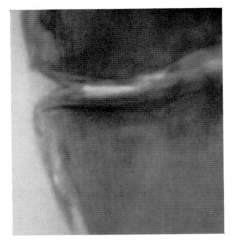
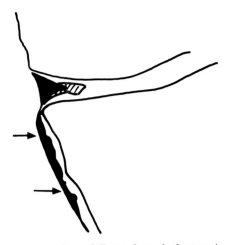

Fig. 178. Lesion of the medial collateral ligament. Liquid contrast medium diffuses through the tear in the capsule distally along the medial tibial plateau (arrows).

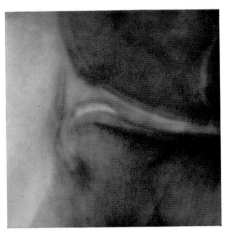
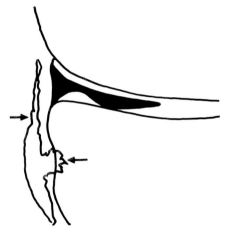

Fig. 179. Scar tissue formation in the bursa semimembranosogastrocnemica (arrows). Irregular contours, signs of shrinking. The bursa is partially filled with contrast medium.

medium or occassionally with air. They are located periarticularly and run in a craniocaudal direction. Their contours are irregular (Fig. 178). Occasionally we can find isolated widening of the menisco-femoral or the menisco-tibial joint space depending on whether the tear is supra- or infra-meniscal (Figs. 180, 181). Medial capsular tears are sometimes seen in connection with a ganglion (Fig. 182). Occasionally we see a meniscus injury on one side combined with a ligamentous injury of the other side.

Tears of the posterior joint capsule not infrequently involve the bursa semimembranoso-

gastrocnemica (Lindblom). They result in deformities of the bursa, irregular contours and changes from scar contractures (Fig. 179; cf. Fig. 64). So far we have not found an arthrogram of a lateral capsular tear in our own material. These tears are relatively rare because the lateral collateral ligament is not firmly attached to the capsule.

b) Lesions of the Cruciate Ligaments

Isolated injuries to the cruciate ligaments are relatively rare and do not usually produce dis

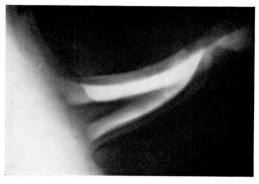
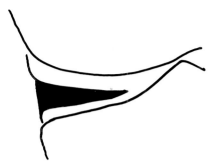

Fig. 180. Lesion of the medial collateral ligament. Infra- and suprameniscal joint spaces are widened (stress film in abduction).

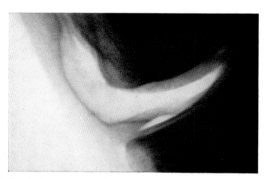
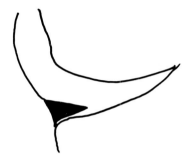

Fig. 181. Lesion of the medial collateral ligament. Only the suprameniscal space is widened (stress film in abduction).

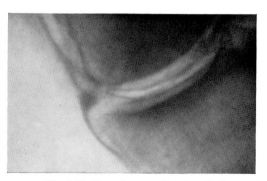
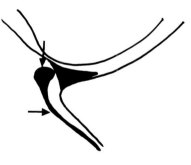

Fig. 182. Capsular ganglion (vertical arrow), with medial capsular tear (horizontal arrow).

turbances of function or lasting symptoms. They are very important, however, in combination with other ligamentous and capsular injuries because the additional loss of a cruciate ligament can increase the instability of the knee considerably. If these lesions produce the characteristic subluxations and "giving way" episodes,

confusion with recurrent meniscal locking is easily possible.

Experience shows that longitudinal tears of the medial meniscus are frequently combined with damage to the anterior cruciate ligament. Careful examination during meniscectomy has revealed damage to the anterior cruciate in up to 20 per cent of all cases (Bircher, Schaer, Smillie, and others). The cause of this high incidence must be found in the mechanism of injury. The anterior cruciate ligament limits internal rotation and anterior displacement of the tibia. Unphysiologic uncontrolled rotatory motions of the knee will damage the cruciate ligament in a similar mechanism, which produces a tear of the meniscus. Smillie has pointed out that an existing meniscus lesion can in itself damage the anterior cruciate ligament. Forceful correction of a flexion deformity from a dislocated bucket-handle tear of the medial meniscus may stretch or tear the anterior cruciate ligament. This can occur during the injury itself, from a forceful attempt to reduce the dislocated portion of the meniscus, or when the patient is permitted to walk on a locked knee for a long period of time.

Forceful abduction of the leg can also produce a tear of the cruciate ligament but only after the medial collateral ligament has been torn completely (Fig. 183).

*Recognition* of a cruciate ligament lesion is often difficult and requires experience. After a fresh injury to the knee joint, examination is usually difficult because of spasm and contracture of musculature and the frequently massive joint effusion. Adequate evaluation of the cruciate ligaments is possible only after aspiration of the effusion under general anesthesia which

should be used much more frequently in the evaluation of fresh unclear knee injuries (Smillie).

The only reliable symptom of a cruciate ligament lesion is the so-called *drawer sign*. The knee is examined in a position of 90 degrees of flexion. A positive drawer sign reveals abnormal anterior or posterior displacement of the tibia in a sagittal direction. It must be pointed out, however, that this displacement is pronounced only in those cases where relaxation or a tear of the medial collateral ligament is present in addition to the cruciate ligament lesion. When the collateral ligament is intact, displacement is frequently only a few millimeters and the cruciate ligament tear is often missed even after careful examination and comparison with the other side. Occasionally routine *X-ray examination* of the knee joint is helpful if a fracture of the tibial spine can be visualized. We have found no fresh cruciate ligament injuries in our series of arthrograms.

According to Lindblom, coagula or edema can lead to a bulging of the anterior cruciate ligament shadow in the *arthrogram*. It should be pointed out that injuries to the anterior cruciate ligament are much more frequent than those of the posterior ligament.

In older lesions the arthrogram frequently reveals absence, irregular contours, or a very small and deformed atrophic cruciate ligament (Fig. 184). According to Palmer an anterior cruciate ligament, which has been torn off its femoral attachment, can be folded over and lie under the infrapatellar fat pad and in front of the tibial attachment of the ligament. The ligament is best visualized on a lateral view of the knee in 45 degrees of flexion and minimal internal rotation. X-rays taken in the anterior drawer position are even more demonstrative.

## 2) Cartilage and Bone Changes

### a) Arthrosis Deformans

Arthrosis deformans plays an important role in the differential diagnosis of a meniscus lesion, mainly because both conditions frequently exist concurrently. Almost all meniscus lesions will produce local damage to the articular cartilage with time and thus lead to secondary arthritic

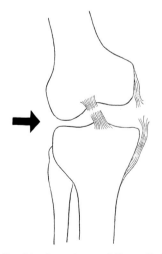

Fig. 183. Combined rupture of the collateral and cruciate ligaments from forced abduction of the leg.

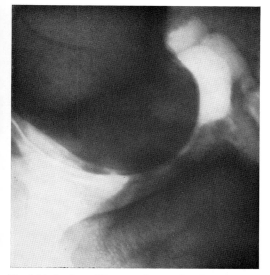
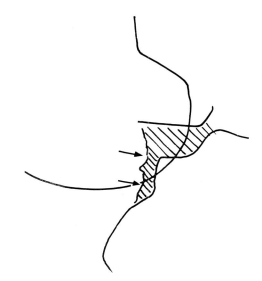

Fig. 184. Lesion of the anterior cruciate ligament. Lateral view in flexion of 45 degrees. The cruciate ligaments are crosshatched. Anterior cruciate ligament shows irregular borders and is markedly narrowed (arrows).

changes. In older patients with advanced degenerative arthritis of the knee, we usually find degenerative changes and small tears in the menisci. Symptoms of degenerative arthritis of the knee are usually not very characteristic. Minor trauma or excessive use of the knee joint will often produce symptoms with recurrent effusions and localized tenderness in the area of the joint space and can very easily be confused with a meniscus lesion, especially when the degenerative arthritis is in its early stage and X-ray changes are only minimal. The presence of spur formation and other arthritic changes on the other hand does not rule out a meniscus lesion.

Thorough diagnostic evaluation is absolutely necessary in these cases, because exploratory arthrotomy in the presence of degenerative changes can produce a severe flare-up of arthritic symptoms. Excision of a torn meniscus, on the other hand, may prevent or retard progression of the degenerative changes to a certain extent. If clinical examination cannot distinguish between the two conditions with enough certainty, *arthrography* is a valuable diagnostic tool. Degenerative arthritis in its beginning stages is usually a chondrosis. Sclerosis of the bone and osteophyte formation usually are secondary

changes. The arthrogram will show cartilaginous changes in their early stages in the form of narrowing and destruction of the articular cartilage (Fig. 185). Secondary localized arthritic changes in the area of a meniscus lesion (Fig. 186) and degenerative changes with tears of the menisci in older patients with advanced arthrosis can frequently be demonstrated in the arthrogram (Fig. 187). Quite often, however, it cannot be determined with certainty whether the meniscus lesion or the degenerative bone and cartilage changes were the primary lesion.

### b) Osteochondritis Dissecans

Osteochondritis dissecans will frequently produce loose bodies in the knee joint and lead to typical locking which can easily be confused with a meniscus lesion. The lesion represents a subchondral avascular necrosis of bone of unknown etiology. Most authors feel that mechanical factors play an important etiological role. A single trauma or frequently repeated microtrauma can lead to local disturbances of nutrition and to fatigue fractures (Buri and Geiser, Gschwend, Mau, Rutishauser, Smillie, and others). The experimental studies of Bandi, Burckhardt, Nagura, and Rehbein appear to confirm this opin-

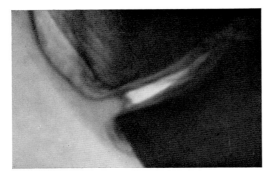

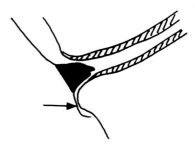

Fig. 185. Arthrosis and meniscus lesion. Stump-like appearance of the meniscus (black), thinning of the articular cartilage (crosshatched). Osteophyte (arrow) on the medial tibial plateau.

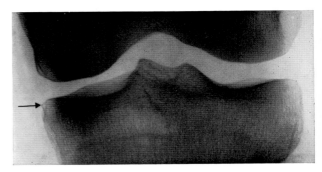

Fig. 186. Secondary arthrosis after meniscus lesion. Nineteen-year-old man. Arthrogram 2 months after accident. Small osteophyte on the medial tibial plateau, which is visible on regular X-ray (right, arrow). Below: Arthrogram. The meniscus is fragmented.

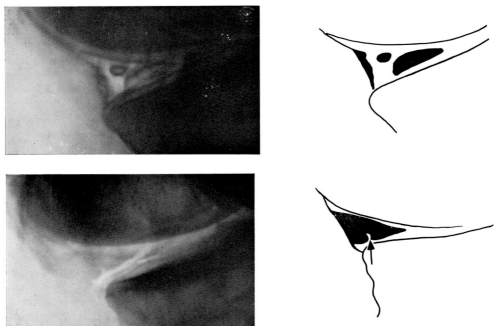

Fig. 187. Primary (?) arthrosis. Sixty-three-year-old man without history of trauma. Generalized arthrosis. Small tear on the undersurface of the plump, degenerated meniscus (arrow).

ion. In addition, constitutional factors seem to play a role. Occasionally several joints are involved simultaneously and familial occurrence has been observed (Zellweger and Ebnöther).

In the knee joint the condition is usually located on the medial femoral condyle and less frequently on the lateral femoral condyle. Detachment of the necrotic cartilage-bone fragment may take several years and the lesion can be asymptomatic for quite some time. Complaints frequently do not occur until the fragment is well demarcated. In the beginning clinical symptoms are not very characteristic and usually consist of diffuse pain, irritation of the knee joint after excessive use, weakness, or a feeling of instability on weight bearing, etc. A trivial injury sometimes produces detachment of the necrotic piece and can lead to typical locking. The loose body can change its position frequently and the clinical picture of the different recurrent locking episodes can vary. The patients frequently observe migration of the joint mouse. Occasionally the loose body can be palpated under the joint capsule.

In most cases diagnosis can be made on a routine *X-ray* of the knee (Fig. 188). As mentioned above, the osteochondritic process is usually localized on the lateral aspect of the medial fem-

oral condyle in the area of the insertion of the posterior cruciate ligament (Köhler-Zimmer). The lateral view usually shows clearly that the lesion is more extensive in the sagittal plane than in the frontal plane. A small step in the articular surface can frequently be seen. The detached bone and cartilage fragment can remain in situ as a "resting mouse" or can be completely detached as a loose body (Köhler-Zimmer), which can be demonstrated by X-rays in two planes.

Occasionally the loose body consists predominantly or entirely of cartilage and then can not be visualized on the routine X-ray. In these cases the *arthrogram* can be of great help. Even small cartilaginous lesions, such as early bulging, beginning detachment, and small cartilage or bone defects, can be visualized quite well on the arthrogram (Fig. 189).

This finding should not be confused with circumscribed cartilaginous lesions in the neighborhood of meniscus tears, which can have a similar appearance (Fig. 190). Osteochondritis dissecans of the patella is a rare lesion. We have observed one case of osteochondritis dissecans on the posterior surface of the patella. This patient also had an extensive lesion of the medial meniscus (Fig. 191).

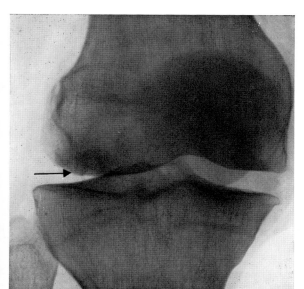

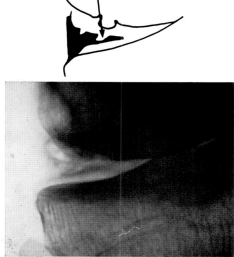

Fig. 188. Osteochondritis dissecans. Left: Regular X-ray, osteocartilaginous lesion visible (arrow). Right: Arthrogram, meniscus lesion.

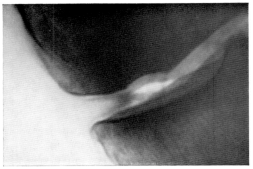
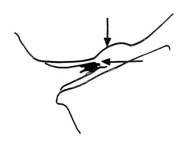

Fig. 189. Osteochondritis dissecans. Small crater (vertical arrow). Meniscus with dull inner border and imbibed with contrast medium. Meniscus lesion (horizontal arrow).

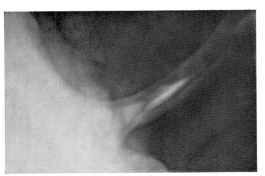

Fig. 190. Osteochondritis dissecans. Small cartilaginous lesion (vertical arrow) adjacent to a meniscus lesion. The meniscus has a dull inner border. Articular cartilage (crosshatched).

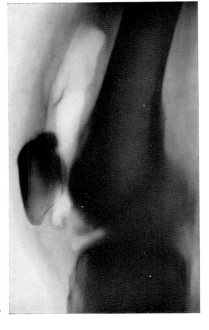

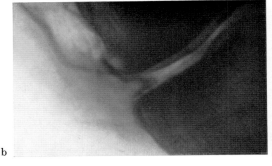

b

a

Fig. 191a. Double-contrast arthrogram, lateral tomogram. Deep crater in the upper half of the articular surface of the patella from osteochondritis dissecans.

Fig. 191b. The same patient has a tear and degeneration of the medial meniscus.

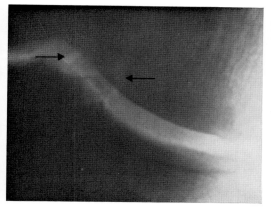
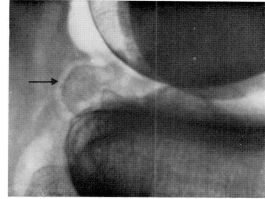

Fig. 192. Osteochondromatosis (air arthrogram). A loose body is seen in the dorso-medial portion of the inferior capsular space. AP view on the left, lateral view on the right. The loose body is delineated by a layer of air (arrows).

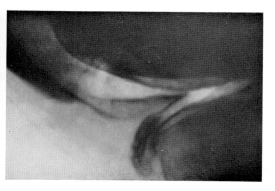

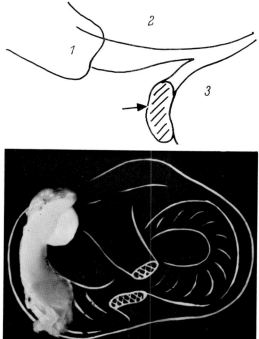

Fig. 193. Osteochondromatosis (double contrast arthrogram). The loose body is seen anteriorly in the inferomedial capsular space. Above: Arthrogram: Area of the anterior horn. 1. Patella. 2. Femur. 3. Tibia. The arrow points to the loose body. Below: Surgical specimen. The medial meniscus had to be removed because the loose body was trapped underneath it.

### c) Osteochondromatosis

Osteochondromatosis or capsular chondromatosis can occur separately or in connection with other degenerative joint diseases. It produces free joint bodies and can lead to typical locking episodes. The lesion consists of small, frequently multiple cartilaginous bodies, which develop in the synovial tissue. They can be pedunculated or float free inside the joint. They frequently grow even after they have been completely detached and can show secondary calcification or ossification.

The etiology of the disease is unknown. The most widely accepted theory is that of a benign tumorous growth of the synovial membrane or tissue metaplasia. According to Anderson the condition represents ectopic cartilage and bone growth because all joint components come from the same embryonic tissue. The condition usually develops in spurts and is not related to trauma. However, the influence of trauma cannot always be excluded.

A *diagnosis* of osteochondromatosis can usually be made from a routine X-ray. The calcified chondromata are usually multiple and vary in size. They are most frequently located in the suprapatellar pouch.

The *arthrogram* will also help to determine whether the calcified body is located intra- or extra-articularly. A simple air arthrogram of the joint without positive contrast medium will often give good results with exact localization of the free bodies (Figs. 192, 193). Purely cartilaginous bodies without calcification can be visualized only with the arthrogram.

### d) Chondromalacia Patellae

Occasionally we must consider chondromalacia of the patella (Haglund-Löwen-Fründ's disease) in our differential diagnosis. The condition represents a painful cartilage degeneration on the articular surface of the patella of unknown etiology. The fact that the patients are usually younger individuals makes the possibility of a constitutional factor very likely. Most authors, however, are of the opinion that the pathologic process is precipitated by a single or sometimes repeated trauma. This produces infraction and disturbance of nutrition in the subchondral bone, which results in cartilaginous changes. Because of the very slow progression of the chondromalacia the original trauma can frequently not be elicited. Symptoms from the original contusion frequently clear up completely. After weeks or months, sometimes years, forceful use of the quadriceps or repeated minor trauma will lead to vague, dull, or sometimes sharp pain inside the joint, which the patient can usually not localize accurately. Occasionally the patient may experience sudden sharp pain without external trauma. These sudden painful episodes can sometimes lead to confusion with a meniscus lesion. The diagnosis of chondromalacia of the patella

is often very difficult. In the early stage of the disease the cartilaginous surface of the patella is still intact and crepitus is absent. Compression of the articular surface of the patella will elicit or increase the pain and this is usually the only diagnostic sign. The patients will frequently experience pain when they walk upstairs in contrast to the complaints from a meniscus lesion which are usually more pronounced when the patient goes downstairs. Pain under the patella when the patient is asked to step on a stool or small chair with his affected leg is a very reliable diagnostic sign. Pain under the patella can also be produced when the knee is moved while the examiner's hand presses the patella against the femoral condyles. Progressive degeneration of the cartilaginous surface of the patella will later produce the characteristic crepitus in the patellofemoral joint which occasionally can be heard from a distance. The irregularity of the articular surface of the patella can best be demonstrated when the patella is moved over the femoral condyles under pressure while the quadriceps muscle is relaxed. Routine *X-ray examination*, especially in early cases, is not very helpful in the diagnosis of chondromalacia of the patella. In advanced cases the lateral X-ray may show an irregular appearance of the posterior surface of the patella (Cave et al.). In the AP view the patella may sometimes appear mottled. Köhler and Zimmer have pointed out that the normal patella of the young patient may occasionally show irregularity of the posterior surface. According to Billing the diagnosis of chondromalacia is likely when marginal osteophytes are present on the patella.

The first pathologic changes in chondromalacia are swelling of the cartilage which then progresses to dessication and thinning of the cartilage with tear formation and destruction. The bone reacts to these changes with osteophyte formation. Swelling of the cartilage, tear formation and narrowing can be shown *arthrographically*, especially in combination with lateral tomograms (Fig. 194). The axial view can also show cartilage changes, irregular contour, and imbibition with liquid contrast medium (Fig. 195). A diagnosis of chondromalacia of the patella from the arthrogram can only be made when marked changes are present. An early diagnosis is not possible

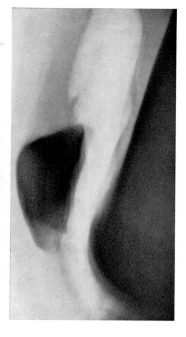
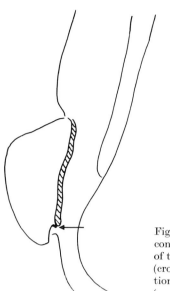

Fig. 194. Lateral tomogram (double contrast arthrogram). Marked thinning of the articular cartilage of the patella (crosshatched) and osteophyte formation on the inferior edge of the patella (arrow). Typical finding with chondromalacia of the patella.

from the arthrogram. It must be made by clinical examination. Osteochondritis dissecans of the patella should be considered in the differential diagnosis. Lavner has described several cases and we have some in our own material (Fig. 191).

## 3) Synovitis and Bursitis

### a) Chronic Synovitis

Chronic irritations and inflammatory processes of the knee joint can very easily simulate a meniscus lesion. This is especially true for the so-called *traumatic synovitis* or *arthritis*. Simple sprains or contusions of the knee joint can lead to persistent infiltrations of the capsule and effusions with thickening and tenderness of the capsular folds. A tender rim is frequently present along the attachment of the menisci which contrary to a meniscus lesion does not disappear inside the joint with flexion. A contracture of the capsule or marked effusion can produce limitation of extension in these cases and only arthrography or exploratory arthrotomy can clarify the diagnosis. The most striking finding in the arthrogram of a knee joint with chronic hydrops is the size of the dilated joint spaces and especially the

bursae. The bursae are more prone to dilatation from an effusion because they are not protected by the strong capsular structures (Fig. 196).

Quite frequently a chronic traumatic synovitis is only a symptom of a *Sudeck's dystrophy* of the

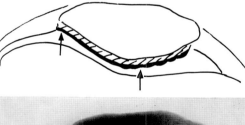
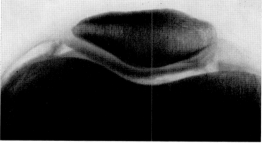

Fig. 195. Chondromalacia of the patella. Axial view of the patella. Double contrast arthrogram. Irregular contour of the articular cartilage of the patella (crosshatched) and imbibition with contrast medium (arrows).

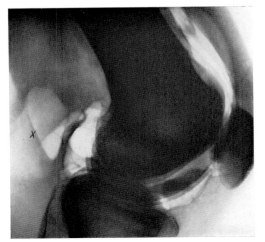

Fig. 196. Chronic effusion of the knee (synovitis exudativa). Widening of the joint spaces is especially striking in the bursa semimembranosogastrocnemica (x).

knee joint. An exploratory arthrotomy to clarify the diagnosis can produce a flare-up of the dystrophic changes. Contrast arthrography is preferable because it is less traumatic. Specific or nonspecific inflammations of the knee joint can occasionally be confused with a meniscus lesion. This can occur with infectious arthritis and in the initial stage of tuberculous arthritis, as pointed out by Ficat and Vuillet. Our own series contains one case of early rheumatoid arthritis

with vague symptoms where arthrography was performed because of suspected meniscus lesion. The arthrogram is shown in Fig. 197. Massive layers of fibrin cover the destroyed meniscus and produce irregular grainy appearance of the synovium. The liquid contrast medium is diluted and permeates the synovial membrane. Marked cartilage destruction is present.

## b) Hoffa's Disease

In 1904 Hoffa described traumatic and inflammatory changes of the infrapatellar fat pad as a clinical entity. This condition is characterized by painful enlargement of the fat pad which is often accompanied by effusion and limitation of function of the knee joint. Entrapment of hypertrophic villi of the fat pad between the condyles can easily simulate a meniscus lesion.

Opinions regarding the incidence and clinical significance of this condition vary in the literature. Most authors agree, however, that Hoffa's disease as a primary independent condition is extremely rare. During arthrotomy of the knee, we frequently find enlargement, reddening and fibrosis of the fatty folds. Schaer found damage to the fat pad in more than 50 per cent of all arthrotomies done for meniscus lesions. According to Groh, damage to the fat pad can be found in 14 per cent of the late changes after ligamentous damage. In most cases these changes are part

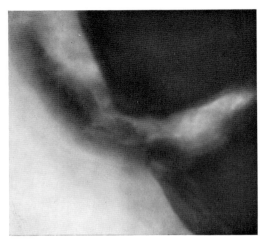
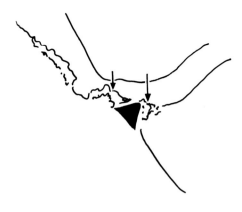

Fig. 197. Arthrogram of patient with rheumatoid polyarthritis (verified by biopsy). Fibrin layers (arrows) partially obscure the destroyed meniscus (black).

of a chronic traumatic synovitis (Buerkle de la Camp). We have only one case in our whole series where locking was produced by trapping of an enlarged fold of the fat pad. We share *Krömer's* opinion that systematic excision of all portions of the fat pad which show pathologic changes is not justified because it increases considerably the risk of postoperative bleeding and effusions. Clinical symptoms of Hoffa's disease are not very characteristic. The complaints are usually produced or increased with strong tension on the patellar ligament, especially when walking downhill. Occasionally the contours of the infrapatellar depressions are less pronounced. Tenderness in the anterior joint space does not change with flexion in contrast to that from a meniscus lesion. Bleeding into the fat pad can occasionally lead to calcifications of varying size and shape and can be seen on routine *X-ray* (Fig. 198). Occasionally small calcifications can be seen in the dorsal fat pad of the knee joint. They probably represent posttraumatic changes. Van de Berg and Crevecoeur have described tears of the dorsal fat pad. Enlarged villi of the fat pad can easily be visualized in the *arthrogram* (Fig. 199). Figure 200 shows changes after partial resection of the fat pad.

*c) Villous Synovitis*

Villous synovitis should not be confused with Hoffa's disease. This condition represents a slowly progressing disease of the entire synovial membrane which extends into the joint with irregular tongues and villi. Occasionally several joints are involved simultaneously or successively. The etiology is uncertain. According to *Anderson*, it is not clear whether the disease represents an inflammatory process or a benign neoplasm. The histologic picture shows masses of granulation tissue with giant cells, lipoid-laden phagocytes, and blood pigment, which is responsible for the dark pigmentation.

Routine *X-rays* show cystoid radiolucent areas inside the bone in the area of the intercondylar fossa (Bessler and Rüttimann) (Fig. 201). In the *arthrogram* the pathologic changes can be differentiated best in the suprapatellar pouch (Fig. 202). Villi and tongues as well as loculated structures are visible within the joint spaces.

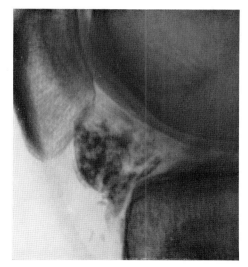

Fig. 198. Extensive calcification of the infrapatellar fat pad.

*d) Diseases of the Bursae*

The bursa of the popliteus muscle can increase in size considerably under the influence of acute or chronic inflammation. Its contents can be emptied into the knee joint. When the bursa is separate, however, it impinges on the lateral posterior joint space from below and produces a typical finding in the arthrogram (Fig. 203).

It does not produce any symptoms which would indicate an arthrogram. Other bursae, such as the bursa semimembranosogastrocnemica, can produce similar signs.

## 4) Ganglia and Tumors

*a) Ganglia of the Menisci*

Ganglia or cysts of the menisci are important because they are prone to tears and can pose similar problems in disability evaluation as do meniscus lesions. The lesion is a multiloculated mucinous degenerative cyst of the meniscus, which frequently involves the joint capsule or permeates it. The patient is usually a young male in the second or third decade. Cysts are much more frequent in the lateral meniscus but ganglia of the medial meniscus have been described. The clinical symptoms are not very characteristic in the beginning. The patient complains of dull

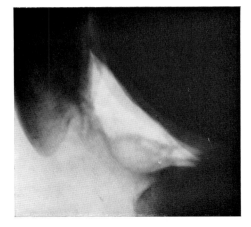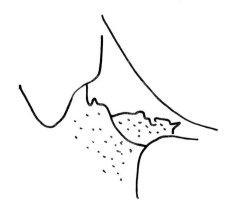

Fig. 199. Infrapatellar fat pad, villous enlargement (dotted).

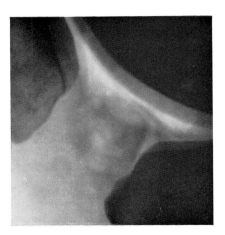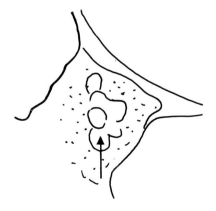

Fig. 200. Status after excision of villi from the infrapatellar fat pad (dotted). Lacunar appearance (arrow)

poorly localized pain in the knee joint, which is precipitated or increased by physical activity. Occasionally a minor contusion or sprain can precipitate the painful episode and trauma is then often made responsible for the development of the ganglion.

Physical examination reveals a firm, elastic swelling at the level of the joint space, but occasionally proximal or distal to it. Small ganglia can only be detected by palpation. A large ganglion of the anterior half of the meniscus can be seen as a small bulge when the knee is in full extension or slight flexion. With further flexion of the knee the bulge usually disappears because the meniscus is displaced into the joint. As the ganglion increases in size it becomes softer and occasionally fluctuation can be shown. A large ganglion quite often produces limitation of motion. This, however, can also be the result of a simultaneous meniscus tear. The roentgen findings of a meniscus ganglion have already been described in the chapter on routine X-ray examination and arthrography of degenerative meniscus lesions (Fig. 135).

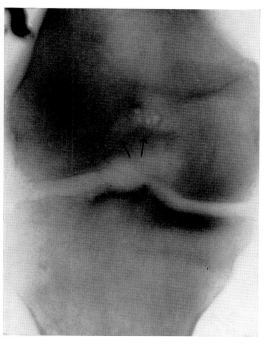

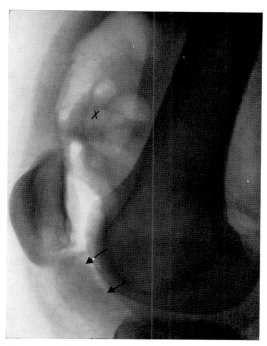

Fig. 201. Tomogram of the right knee joint of an 18-year-old female with villous synovitis. Multiple small cystic lesions are seen in the roof of the inter-condylar fossa.

Fig. 202. Villous synovitis. Formation of villi and septa is visualized well in the suprapatellar pouch (X), giving a loculated appearance. Note the enlarged infrapatellar fat pad (arrows).

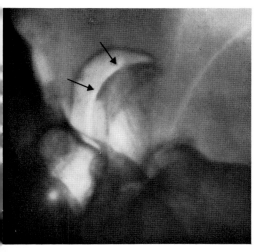

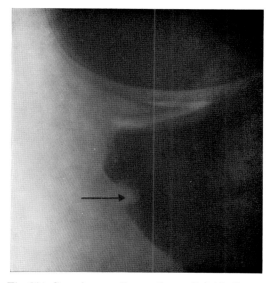

Fig. 203. Popliteal bursitis. The enlarged popliteal bursa compresses the posterior portion of the medial joint space and gives it a concave contour (arrows).

Fig. 204. Capsular ganglion on the medial side. Large erosion on the medial tibial plateau (arrow).

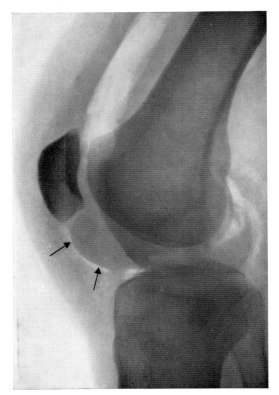

Fig. 205. Giant-cell tumor of the knee joint (air arthrogram). Sharply delineated crescent-shaped tumor shadow in the anterior joint compartment (arrows) (Catolla).

### b) Ganglia of the Capsule

Cystic changes can not only arise from the menisci but also from the joint capsule. These can usually be palpated on the lateral side of the knee joint as a firm, rather immobile and slightly tender structure. The routine *X-ray* occasionally shows a small circumscribed defect below the tibial plateau (Fig. 204).

The arthrogram does not show any changes because the ganglion is located extra-articularly, distal and lateral to the tibial plateau.

### c) Tumors of the Knee Joint

Tumors in the area of the knee joint are rare and do not play a significant role in the differential diagnosis of meniscus lesions. They can arise from the joint capsule or from the menisci and can produce locking or limitation of motion depending on their location. The literature describes fibromata, chondromata, hemangiomata, giant cell tumors, etc. (Henschen, Ritter, Tobler). Figure 205 shows an xanthomatous giant cell tumor, which presents itself in the arthrogram as a soft tissue shadow in the anterior joint space. We are indebted to Catolla for permission to use this case.

CHAPTER 7

# Therapeutic Problems

The literature on meniscus lesions in the last few years has been voluminous, but opinions as to the best and most efficient method of treatment for the damaged meniscus vary considerably. The main reason for this probably stems from the fact that early results after meniscectomy do not give us the complete answer and that a follow-up of 10 or 20 years is necessary for a long term evaluation of our results. Unfortunately no large series with long follow-ups

exists at the present time. Some guidelines of a more general nature, however, seem to be universally accepted today and will be discussed here.

1) The menisci are important structures of the knee joint and are necessary for normal function. They enlarge the weight-bearing surface of the joint and act as elastic cushions to distribute the pressure more evenly. Their absence increases stress on the articular cartilage and en-

hances development of arthritic changes. Resection of a meniscus should therefore be done only with strict indications.

2) The damaged meniscus irritates the joint and will eventually lead to damage of the articular cartilage and thus to irreversible arthritic changes. Damaged menisci which cause symptoms, irritation and locking should be removed.

3) The diagnosis should be clarified preoperatively, if at all possible, with the help of history, clinical findings, and if necessary, arthrography of the joint. Exploratory arthrotomy permits only a limited examination of the joint, and damage to the undersurface of the posterior horn and the opposite meniscus is easily overlooked. Exploratory arthrotomy can occasionally aggravate a coexisting condition.

4) The operative technic for resection of the damaged meniscus should be meticulous and should spare ligaments, capsule, and articular cartilage to permit optimal conditions for regeneration of the meniscus.

## 1) Indications for Conservative and Operative Therapy

A damaged meniscus should be removed only if it causes typical complaints or disturbance of function. This opinion is shared by most surgeons today. Once we have made a diagnosis of a meniscus lesion with the necessary certainty, there is no sense in postponing the procedure. The patient will suffer unnecessary loss of time and income and will sooner or later come to operation anyhow. Experience of the surgical clinic in Zurich shows that the results of meniscectomy are better when the interval between trauma and operation is short. Late arthritic changes are less severe after early operation (Ritzmann).

Not all meniscus lesions, however, require immediate surgery. The indications for conservative and operative treatment will be discussed in subsequent chapters on the basis of Groh's classification.

### a) Fresh Traumatic Tears

We have already mentioned in the chapter on pathogenesis of meniscus lesions that the first trauma to a histologically "healthy" meniscus will most frequently lead to a partial tear or detachment from the capsule. If the injury is limited to the well vascularized outer zone, healing is possible with conservative therapy. This means that especially in young patients under 20 to 25 years of age, who have not developed degenerative changes of their menisci, conservative treatment can be tried. Combined injuries to the ligamentous structures and the menisci can also be an indication for conservative treatment. Usually the symptoms of the ligamentous injury predominate in the beginning and it is often impossible to detect a concomitant injury to the meniscus with enough certainty. In most cases it is therefore advantageous to treat the ligamentous injury conservatively. Partial detachments of the medial meniscus with ruptures of the medial collateral ligament frequently heal with adequate immobilization.

After the first traumatic episode a good number of patients will become symptom-free with conservative treatment. If locking of the knee joint is present immediately, or if characteristic signs of a meniscus injury are still present after the acute symptoms have subsided, operative treatment is indicated.

Fractures of the tibial plateau are frequently associated with a meniscus injury. As mentioned previously, each compression fracture of the tibial plateau with step formation can lead to a tear or a detachment of the meniscus. These meniscus lesions can later give rise to symptoms and disturbance of functions. Most authors today agree that fractures of the tibial plateau should be treated surgically to insure anatomical reduction and satisfactory late results. Operative reduction also permits us to inspect the joint and remove the torn meniscus.

### b) Late Changes Following Traumatic Tears

When the original injury produces a tear in the avascular inner zone of the meniscus or when immobilization was inadequate for proper healing, the patient will experience new symptoms after a certain period of time. The original tear will gradually become larger and the cartilaginous substance in the region of the tear will gradually degenerate. In contrast to fresh injuries, healing of an old lesion is practically impossible to achieve with conservative therapy, and operation is the treatment of choice.

The patient with a *bucket-handle tear* will give a typical history. He usually tells us that he sustained a knee injury sometime ago and then experienced locking episodes with gradually increasing frequency. There is no question that operative treatment is the method of choice under these circumstances.

In those cases where it is necessary to postpone surgery for good reasons, an attempt to reduce the dislocated meniscus fragment is indicated. This attempt, however, is not always successful and can lead to additional damage to the knee joint if manipulation is not done carefully. In cases where history and clinical findings are less characteristic, the decision to operate can be very difficult. Krömer recommends waiting under these circumstances to see whether the meniscus lesion will extend and produce locking of the joint. We prefer to try to clarify the diagnosis by arthrography when the diagnosis is not clear clinically. We always recommend surgical treatment when the arthrogram shows a definite meniscus tear. When the arthrogram is negative, we prefer to wait.

### c) Spontaneous Detachment (Meniscopathy)

We advocate the same management for those meniscus lesions which develop on the basis of pathologic degeneration rather than traumatic damage. When typical symptoms of a meniscus tear are present, surgical treatment is indicated. This group also comprises patients with persistent or recurrent knee symptoms which are not typical for a meniscus tear and where the history does not reveal any trauma or locking. These symptoms are usually produced by a degenerated and frayed meniscus where the fragments are not large enough to produce locking. The arthrogram will show characteristic changes in patients with meniscopathy in the form of imbibition with contrast medium, fraying or bulging because of cyst formation, etc. (See Figs. 129 to 132.)

Patients with meniscopathy will frequently show other joint changes such as arthritic cartilage and bone lesions, residuals of an osteochondritis dissecans, chondromalacia of the patella, Hoffa's disease, etc. This frequently produces additional diagnostic difficulties and the physician has to evaluate individually whether the majority of the symptoms is due to the meniscus lesion or the degenerative joint changes. When arthritic changes are present in the knee the decision to operate should be made with great care because the trauma of the operation can occasionally produce a flare-up of the arthritis. When there is clear evidence of pathologic changes in the meniscus, we recommend removal of the damaged meniscus because it can enhance progression of the arthritis.

### d) Late Changes in Unstable Joints

In a patient with an unstable knee the meniscus lesion is only part of the generalized degenerative changes produced by the joint instability. The same guide lines as those given for degenerative arthritis apply here. In many cases a well developed musculature can compensate for ligamentous laxity. Operative intervention, however, will frequently produce marked muscle atrophy with impaired stability of the knee. Meniscectomy in the presence of ligamentous instability should be carried out only after careful evaluation and should be combined with ligamentous repair if at all possible. Postoperatively, an intensive quadriceps program is of utmost importance.

## 2) Conservative Treatment

Conservative treatment of the meniscus lesion should always be guided by the clinical findings. If a meniscus lesion after *fresh trauma to the knee joint* is suspected but cannot be confirmed, we usually immobilize the joint in a position of moderate flexion for a few days or apply a compression dressing with plastic sponges and elastic bandages. A significant effusion should be evacuated, repeatedly if necessary. This will make the patient more comfortable and will prevent stretching of the joint capsule which often causes prolonged posttraumatic irritation of the knee joint. After the acute symptoms have subsided, it must be decided whether *plaster immobilization* of the joint should be continued or whether gradual mobilization and weight bearing is indicated. Only a small percentage of fresh meniscus tears will heal with plaster immobilization for 4 to 6 weeks. We, therefore, recommend plaster treatment only in patients with concomitant ligamentous lesions or in young individuals, where the prognosis for healing of the meniscus lesion is much better. The patient should be placed on systematic quadriceps training during plaster immobilization to avoid significant muscle atrophy. These exercises are done in a supine position. The leg is raised off the table approximately 20 to 30 cm. and moved in a circular motion. The exercise should be repeated several times daily for 10 to 15 minutes. The weight of the plaster adds to the load.

When plaster fixation is not indicated, the patient can begin with careful active exercises several days after the injury. Some limitation of extension which may be present in the beginning usually disappears within a short time. Passive stretching to overcome limitation of motion is contraindicated. It can produce considerable irritation of the knee and infiltration of the capsule which impairs motion even more. Manual stretching in the presence of a locked meniscus can also produce damage to the ligamentous structures.

*Quadriceps training* should be started early with isometric exercises of the extended leg. They should be supplemented with gradually increasing resistive exercises after the irritation has cleared up. Whirlpool baths and moist packs to the knee can be added to this treatment but massage and hot air treatment are useless. As soon as the patient is permitted to bear weight on the involved leg, the joint should be bandaged with an elastic bandage. Older patients will frequently benefit from an Unna's paste boot to the leg. The elastic bandage will prevent formation of recurrent effusions to a certain degree and will give the patient additional security when he walks.

*Locking of the knee* from a bucket-handle tear of the meniscus represents a special therapeutic problem. Most surgeons today disapprove of forceful manipulations to reduce the dislocated meniscus because of the risk of producing additional joint damage. We believe that in certain cases careful manipulation can be tried. This is true especially when there is considerable limitation of extension, which makes walking practically impossible. In the mountains, where it is difficult to transport the patient, manual reduction of the locked meniscus can give the patient significant relief and make it possible for him to move his knee through a complete range of motion without much discomfort. Manual reduction of the locking can also be tried for older tears and recurrent locking.

In some cases reduction is possible with simple traction in the longitudinal axis of the leg. Reduction of the dislocated meniscus can be facilitated by distraction of the involved joint spaces. Not infrequently the patient states that occasionally he is able to unlock his knee in this manner either alone or with the help of others.

The method described by *Kulka* is even less traumatic. The patient is asked to let the injured leg hang over the edge of the table or the bed with the knee flexed 90 degrees. This produces relaxation of the musculature and the locked meniscus frequently slides back into its bed spontaneously after a few minutes. This can be facilitated by mild rotatory motions and careful traction in the axis of the leg.

*Smillie* recommends careful rotation of the foot internally or externally with the knee in marked flexion depending on whether the medial or lateral meniscus is injured. This is followed by sudden extension of the knee to reduce the locked meniscus.

When these manipulations are unsuccessful and the patient is in the hospital, one can try reduction of the locking under a short general anesthesia. This procedure may make it difficult to determine whether the locking has been removed because with good relaxation of the musculature the sliding back of the meniscus is frequently difficult to palpate. We must emphasize again that forceful manipulations are contraindicated and that forceful extension of the knee joint against resistance may damage the anterior cruciate ligament.

Occasionally a patient with moderate symptoms may refuse operation. These patients should be instructed in an intensive muscle exercise program because the quadriceps rapidly atrophies in the presence of a symptomatic meniscus lesion. The incidence of recurrent locking can sometimes be reduced by wearing a tight bandage or a knee pad of felt or leather. Without operative treatment, these patients will usually be disabled enough to force them to discontinue all sports activities.

## 3) Operative Treatment

Even though meniscectomy today is a standard procedure and one of the most frequent orthopedic operations, it should only be carried out with proper technic when the indication is clear. The advent of antibiotic therapy has not eliminated postoperative infections and the danger of a hospital-acquired staphylococcal infection is still present. Experience has shown that prophylactic treatment with antibiotics does not prevent postoperative wound infections and cannot take the place of thorough aseptic technic.

The operation should be done carefully and with minimal damage to soft tissues, joint capsule, ligaments, and articular cartilage. Orientation inside the knee joint is often difficult for the unexperienced and damage to the articular surface of the knee can easily occur when the meniscus is excised. These lesions in the articular cartilage can later produce severe arthritic changes. Experience, adequate exposure and the proper instruments are important prerequisites for prevention of these damages.

Operative technic varies from one hospital to another and from one surgeon to another. The following is a description of our own technic which we have used for the last several years. We will also discuss some of the more controversial questions of operative treatment.

### a) Partial or Total Meniscectomy

An important question, one which is asked very frequently, is how much of the injured meniscus should be resected. Most surgeons (Buerkle de la Camp, De Palma, Nicolet, Smillie, Wachsmuth, Watson-Jones, and many others) recommend total excision of the meniscus. Böhler and his school, on the other hand, excise only the torn part of the cartilage. The whole problem is intimately connected with the question of meniscus regeneration. The advocates of partial resection are of the opinion that we cannot always count on regeneration of the meniscus after total meniscectomy. They argue that regenerated cartilage is not true hyaline cartilage. The tissue is of inferior quality and cannot serve as adequate functional replacement for the original meniscus.

From many reoperations and control arthrograms there can be no question, however, but that the meniscus does regenerate (Becker, Bircher, Courvoisier, Landolt, Mandl, Morel, Nicolet, De Oliveira, Rutscheidt, Schaefer, Smillie, etc.). We shall discuss one of our own cases in more detail later.

The fact that the meniscus regenerates after resection is no surprise because any tissue defect in any part of the human body will heal by scar formation (Schaer). The regenerated meniscus is usually somewhat smaller than the original cartilage and shows more fibrous tissue. Occasionally the new meniscus is difficult to distinguish from a normal meniscus either macroscopically or microscopically. In favorable cases we can therefore expect a good functional and morphologic replacement of the meniscus. Regeneration, however, will occur only from the well-vascularized outer zone of the meniscus or the joint capsule but not from a partially resected avascular and degenerated cartilage.

It is usually quite difficult during operation to assess the extent of the degenerative changes. In primary degeneration the entire avascular inner zone is usually involved. After a traumatic tear, the originally healthy cartilage surrounding the tear rapidly develops degenerative changes. When the meniscus is only partially resected, segments of the meniscus with degenerative changes frequently remain in the joint and can later lead to new ruptures and symptoms.

The most important argument for total resection of the meniscus in our opinion is the fact that a small incision over the anterior joint line will not permit a thorough examination of the entire meniscus. Partial tears of the undersurface and small longitudinal tears in the posterior horn are usually visualized only after the meniscus has been excised. Removal of the anterior horn alone will lead almost automatically to new symptoms following surgery. We have seen a number of patients in the last few years where a second operation was necessary for resection of a posterior horn, which was left behind during the original surgery. The following is a discussion of a typical example, which also points out some of the problems of meniscus regeneration.

### H. S. SUVA-No. VII/2724/58

The patient is an asthenic white male who works as a machinist. He underwent meniscectomy of the lateral meniscus of his left knee after locking episodes following a sprain of the knee. Postoperatively he was asymptomatic for 3 years. In 1956 he fell on the ice and sustained an injury to the left knee which was followed by similar complaints on the medial side of the joint. The anterior horn of the medial meniscus was resected elsewhere. After a fall downstairs in 1958 typical locking episodes recurred. The arthrogram revealed a large posterior horn remnant of the medial meniscus with a partial tear (Fig. 206). Increasing symptoms, especially with flexion of the knee, made a third arthrotomy necessary in 1959. Inspection of the joint during operation revealed a smooth shining regenerated segment of 5 mm. width in the anterior half of the medial joint compartment. The posterior horn was flattened, frayed and partially detached from the capsule. Total resection of the remaining posterior horn and the regenerate was performed. Microscopically the posterior horn revealed massive fatty and mucinous degeneration. The regenerated segment consisted of fibrocartilage and showed minor fatty degeneration in several areas.

The patient was asymptomatic during the following 3 years. In February of 1962 he fell and injured his knee on a sharp corner. A persistent painful swelling developed in the area of the patellar fat pad and the patient complained of locking episodes on extension which he localized under the patella. Conservative therapy and intra-articular cortisone injections gave only temporary relief. Routine X-ray examination showed normal joint contours and no loose bodies. With a tentative diagnosis of Hoffa's disease the knee joint was opened for the fourth time. Operation revealed a markedly enlarged and reddened infrapatellar fat pad with two long hyalinized villi, which even under anesthesia were caught between the patella and the femoral condyle when the joint was extended. The joint surfaces were smooth and did not show any arthritic changes. A small well-circumscribed area of frayed cartilage was present on the medial border of the articular surface of the patella. In place of the twice resected medial meniscus, a small whitish band of tissue had formed.

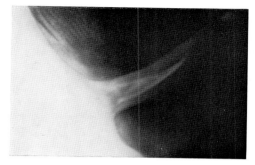

Fig. 206. Status after resection of the anterior horn of the medial meniscus. The arthrogram shows a torn posterior horn with floating fragment.

Inspection of the lateral side revealed a shiny, smooth, regenerated segment of approximately 8 mm. width, which was difficult to distinguish from a normal meniscus. The enlarged villi were resected and the patient went back to work 6 weeks later. He has been asymptomatic ever since.

At present there is no statistical evidence in favor of partial versus total resection. Late results reported in the literature cannot be compared because the guide lines for evaluation differ widely. *Landolt* has recently reported a series of 80 cases, 8 to 12 years after operation, and found that the results after total resection were slightly better than those after partial resection. The small number of cases and the relatively short follow-up period do not allow any definite conclusions.

Our own experience has convinced us that it is better to resect the entire avascular part of the meniscus, including the anterior and especially the posterior horn. It is not necessary to resect the well-vascularized outer zone of the meniscus if it appears intact and is not detached from the capsule. The vascularized peripheral zone forms a good basis for regeneration of the meniscus and can, if necessary, perform the function of a meniscus at least partially if no regeneration should take place. The vascularized outer zone of the meniscus comprises approximately one-third of the width of the meniscus. It can usually be distinguished during surgery by a slight difference in color. Most authors today consider the so-called two-thirds resection of the meniscus as the method of choice (Krömer, Nicolet, Wachs-

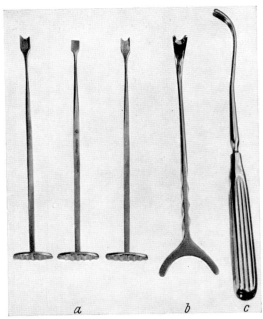

Fig. 207. Instruments: Meniscotomes with guarded cutting surface. a) Smillie. b) Bircher. c) Streli.

horn than to attempt total resection and produce severe and irreversible damage to the joint cartilage. Leaving the posterior horn can be justified when arthrography has shown it to be intact.

### b) Instruments

A great number of instruments have been devised to facilitate resection of the meniscus. Almost every hospital owns a number of specially modified meniscotomes. They usually show a curvature or angulation in their cutting portion to facilitate excision of the crescent-shaped meniscus. It is, of course, possible to resect the meniscus with a normal straight scalpel but damage to the articular cartilage is difficult to avoid, especially if resection is done through a small incision over the anterior joint line. This is also true for all tenotome-like instruments whose cutting surface is unprotected.

We have used the meniscotomes designed by *Smillie* for many years (Figs. 207a and 208a and b). The straight knife is used to detach the easily visualized middle portion of the meniscus. The curved C-shaped knives are protected by two blunt horns, which minimize the risk of damage to the articular cartilage. The longer of the two horns should always remain in contact with the tibial plateau.

Detachment of the posterior horn from the posterior capsule is occasionally facilitated by use of the meniscotomes designed by *Streli* and *Bircher*, which are constructed according to

muth, etc.). We must mention, however, that resection of the entire meniscus including the posterior horn is frequently much more difficult technically than resection of the detached part alone. Experience and careful surgical technic are necessary to avoid damage to the articular cartilage. For the unexperienced, it is usually better to perform a partial resection of the meniscus and leave a portion of the posterior

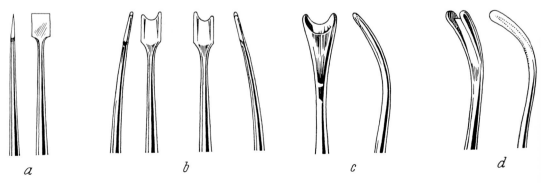

Fig. 208. Detailed view of meniscotomes with guarded cutting surface. a) Smillie's straight knife-like meniscotome. b) Smillie meniscotome, slightly curved. c) Bircher meniscotome with marked curvature. d) Streli meniscotome with marked curvature.

similar principles, but have a larger curvature (Figs. 207 b and c, and 208 c and d). A meniscus forceps with several strong teeth in its anterior portion, small angulated retractors of different length and width, and several regular scissors, forceps, and scalpels complete the instrument set (Fig. 209).

### c) Preparation for Surgery

We have already mentioned that the use of antibiotics should not lead us to neglect the principles of aseptic technic. Purulent infections, pyodermia, and furuncles are strict contraindications to arthrotomy. Meniscectomy is never an emergency operation and should be delayed if conditions are not optimal.

In the last few years we have used hexachlorophene (PhisoHex, Winthrop) for preparation of the skin. The patient is given a complete bath and the skin of the operative field is shaved. A foam of hexachlorophene is then applied to the operative field on the evening before operation and covered with sterile gauze. We have found this procedure to be valuable for all our orthopedic procedures. We prefer hexachlorophene to the alcohol dressings used by us earlier because it is well tolerated and has a long-lasting effect.

### d) Anesthesia

Most surgeons today prefer general anesthesia to local or spinal anesthesia. An experienced surgeon will rarely take longer than 20 to 30 minutes for the procedure and a modern short-acting narcotic, such as pentothal in combination with nitrous oxide or fluothane, is usually adequate. Only in those cases where another procedure, such as ligamentous repair, is planned in addition to meniscectomy, will duration of the operation be prolonged and intubation may be indicated.

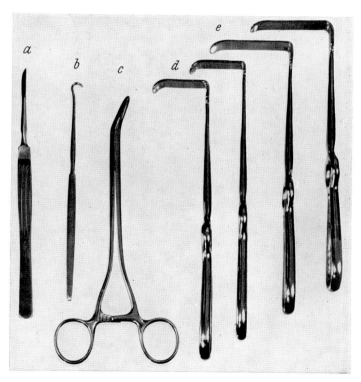

Fig. 209. Instruments: a) Scalpel. b) Meniscus hook. c) Meniscus forceps. d and e) Small Langenbeck retractors of different size.

### e) *Positioning and Tourniquet Control*

Most surgeons today perform the operation under tourniquet control. This produces a bloodless operative field and permits rapid and careful technic with minimal risk of inadvertent joint damage or postoperative infection.

One must realize, however, that interruption of blood supply at the thigh harbors a certain risk of ischemic tissue damage and pressure damage to nerves. The peroneal nerve is especially vulnerable. Application of a tourniquet requires great care and should not be left to an inexperienced attendant. Only soft rubber bandages or padded inflatable cuffs should be used. *After 75 minutes* the tourniquet should be released. Disturbance of arterial circulation on the basis of arteriosclerosis is a strict contraindication to the use of a tourniquet.

Meniscectomy is performed by most surgeons with the knee flexed 90 degrees and the leg hanging over the edge of the table. This permits a maximum of mobility of the leg with a minimum of assistance. After disinfection of the skin the operative field is covered with a sterile plastic sheet, which is glued to the skin with plastic spray or Mastix solution. This eliminates any contact with the skin and does not interfere with orientation.

### f) *Incision*

The incision must permit good exposure and visualization of the operative field, but must avoid all important structures such as tendons, ligaments and nerves. A thorough preoperative work-up will clarify the diagnosis in most cases and will avoid extensive exploratory arthrotomy. Only a small incision of 3–4 cm. length is necessary for the resection of a torn meniscus and the evaluation of the adjacent cartilaginous surfaces, the anterior cruciate ligament, and the infrapatellar fat pad.

Of the many incisions which have been described for meniscectomy, we prefer a small oblique incision over the anterior joint space

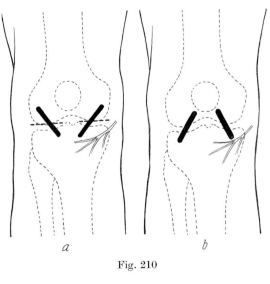

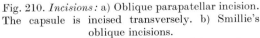

Fig. 210

Fig. 210. *Incisions:* a) Oblique parapatellar incision. The capsule is incised transversely. b) Smillie's oblique incisions.
Fig. 211. Incisions for simultaneous joint exploration in front and behind the collateral ligament: a) DePalma's incision. b) Cave's incision. c) Fisher's incision. d) Jewstropow's incision.

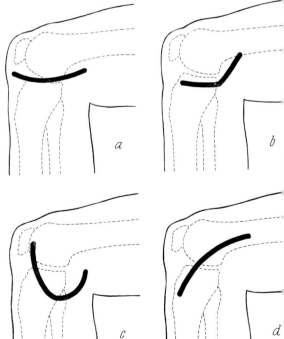

Fig. 211

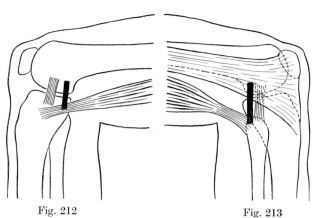

Fig. 212. Separate approach to the posterior horn of the medial meniscus (Smillie)
Fig. 213. Separate approach to the posterior horn of the lateral meniscus.

Fig. 212                                    Fig. 213

Fig. 210a). The skin incision is made in a parapatellar fashion on a line between the femoral condyle and the tibial tubercle. It should not extend too far anteriorly to avoid later discomfort from the scar when kneeling. Care must be taken not to injure the infrapatellar branch of the saphenous nerve in the subcutaneous tissue. The nerve lies over the tendon of the sartorius muscle, crosses the joint in the area of the medial collateral ligament and goes to the tibial tubercle. The skin incision is usually made approximately one fingerbreadth proximal to the nerve. Fascia and joint capsule are incised in the transverse direction approximately 1 to 1.5 cm. above the tibial plateau. The base of the meniscus must not be touched by the incision. If necessary the capsular incision can be extended to the collateral ligament.

Smillie has recommended an incision that runs in the opposite direction (Fig. 210b). The oblique incision begins at the inferior pole of the patella and extends laterally to the tibial plateau. Skin and capsule are incised in the same direction. The incision divides the fibrous capsule in the direction of its fibers and avoids injury to the infrapatellar fat pad. However, the risk of injuring the infrapatellar branch of the saphenous nerve and the base of the meniscus is much greater.

Occasionally, resection of the posterior horn can present difficulties. Several authors have therefore recommended incisions which permit simultaneous exposure of the joint anterior and posterior to the collateral ligament (Fig. 211).

Division of the collateral ligament to facilitate exposure, as recommended recently by Jewstropow, Mommsen, and others, is a risky procedure and in our opinion completely unnecessary. It complicates the operation and postoperative treatment and should be avoided. In those cases where the anterior incision alone is inadequate, we prefer to open the joint through a second smaller incision in the posterior joint space (Figs. 212 and 213). This procedure rarely, if ever, produces additional trauma to the joint.

The sartorius muscle is encountered on the medial side after incision of skin and subcutaneous tissue and should be retracted dorsally. Care must be taken not to injure the saphenous nerve. The joint capsule, which is relaxed in the position of flexion, can easily be identified between the medial collateral ligament and the gastrocnemius tendon, which sometimes must be detached partially. The joint capsule is incised transversely.

The approach on the lateral side is somewhat more complicated. The head of the fibula with the insertion of the lateral collateral ligament and the long biceps tendon serves as a guide line. The skin and subcutaneous tissue are incised longitudinally and the iliotibial tract exposed. The iliotibial tract is separated from the biceps tendon and retracted anteriorly. This exposes the round lateral collateral ligament. Next, the lateral head of the gastrocnemius is exposed and detached from the joint capsule. A transverse incision of the joint capsule gives good exposure of the posterior joint space and the posterior horn of the meniscus. Inspection of the anterior half of the joint through this incision is obscured by the popliteal tendon, which lies under the lateral collateral ligament.

### g) Technic of Resection

Before we enter into a detailed discussion of meniscus resection, we would like to emphasize that a small incision is adequate only when it is placed in a parapatellar location just above the tibial plateau. We prefer to use plastic draping, which does not interfere with orientation. Even then the unexperienced may have occasional difficulties locating the joint space, especially in adipose patients. The use of a long needle will help considerably in locating the articular surface of the tibia. Synovium and capsule are only a few millimeters thick over the femoral condyle, and the capsular incision is best started there. If the incision is started farther distally it can easily be carried into the infrapatellar fat pad with damage to its blood vessels which may lead to troublesome postoperative bleeding.

Next, two blunt retractors are inserted into the inner and outer edge of the wound and the excess synovial fluid is removed from the joint cavity.

Inspection of the joint is facilitated by exerting traction on the inferior capsular edge by means of a small, sharp hook. It is important to note all operative findings (i.e., quantity and color of the synovial fluid, condition of the joint capsule, infrapatellar fat pad, articular surfaces and ligaments, etc.) accurately in the operative report. These findings may be important for prognosis and subsequent disability evaluation. Inspection of the menisci must be done with extreme care. Total longitudinal tears and injuries to the anterior horn are usually detected without difficulty. Quite frequently, however, the anterior portion of the meniscus appears intact. Strong abduction or adduction in combination with internal or external rotation of the leg will usually make it possible to visualize the free inner border of the posterior horn. Tongue-shaped tears of the posterior portion of the meniscus can usually be detected in this manner. A detachment or longitudinal tear of the posterior horn, or partial tears on the undersurface, are very difficult to

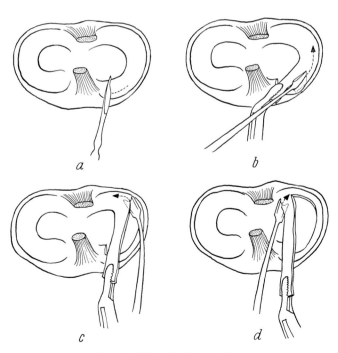

*a*          *b*

*c*          *d*

Fig. 214. Technic of resection.

visualize. One can try to palpate the meniscus carefully with a small, blunt hook or a special meniscus probe. If no abnormal findings are detected, despite thorough examination, the surgeon faces a difficult decision. A seemingly intact meniscus may well lead to a second arthrotomy at a later date because a lesion was overlooked. We feel that the meniscus should always be removed when clinical symptoms or arthrographic findings are indicative of a meniscus lesion. Quite often a lesion in the posterior horn will not become apparent until after removal of the meniscus. In those cases where arthrography was not performed and preoperative clinical findings were questionable, especially as far as localization of the lesion is concerned, it is advisable to inspect the entire joint. Adequate retraction of the medial incision will permit inspection of the anterior cruciate ligament, the infrapatellar fat pad and the anterior one-third of the lateral meniscus. It is the lesser evil to make an additional lateral incision when a lesion of the lateral meniscus is suspected than to remove an intact medial meniscus and leave the injured lateral meniscus behind.

Traction on the inferior edge of the capsule will permit good visualization of the anterior half of the meniscus. The meniscus is incised in a transverse direction approximately 3 mm. from the capsule and as close as possible to its insertion in the area of the eminentia intercondylaris (Fig. 214a). The anterior horn is then grasped with a forceps and pulled out of the wound. Insertion of a blunt retractor between the capsule and/or the collateral ligament and the femoral condyle will permit good visualization of the middle one-third of the meniscus. This portion of the meniscus is detached with a straight, sharp meniscotome (Fig. 214b). Detachment of the posterior horn is the most difficult phase of the procedure and should always be done with the necessary care. Strong traction is applied to the meniscus by means of a forceps and the curved meniscotome is inserted into the plane of resection with the longer of its two horns in contact with the articular surface of the tibia (Fig. 214c). The meniscotome is then carefully advanced around the femoral condyle. In those cases where the curvature of the Smillie menis-

cotome is inadequate, we prefer to use the instrument developed by *Streli* which has a greater curve. Strong traction will displace the meniscus into the intercondylar notch after adequate detachment has been obtained. The joint space is then opened with the knee in moderate flexion. This will permit visualization of the posterior portion of the eminentia intercondylaris. Visualization of the posterior horn is occasionally even better with the knee in extreme flexion. Smillie's curved meniscotome is then introduced into the intercondylar fossa between the anterior cruciate ligament and the femoral condyle and the posterior horn of the meniscus detached (Fig. 214d). The area of resection of the posterior horn is then thoroughly inspected and fibers and cartilaginous threads which were left behind are removed. There is very little difference between the technic of resection for the medial and lateral meniscus. Detachment of the posterior horn of the lateral meniscus may be somewhat easier because the meniscus is more mobile and inserts more ventrally. The resection of a *bucket-handle tear* depends on the width of the detached portion of the meniscus. Frequently this consists of two-thirds or even the entire width of the meniscus. Resection of the bucket-handle alone is sufficient in these cases (Fig. 215c). If the peripheral portion of the meniscus is wide, irregular or fragmented, we prefer to resect the entire menis-

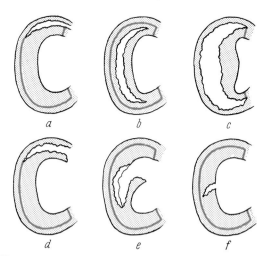

Fig. 215. Technic of two-thirds resection for different tears.

cus and leave only a small capsular rim (Fig. 215b). We follow the same procedure for partial longitudinal tears, detachments of the anterior or posterior horn and for circumscribed pedunculated ruptures or transverse tears. In all these cases we perform the classical two-thirds resection of the meniscus (Figs. 215a, d, e, and f).

Occasionally one encounters *difficulties when resecting a meniscus*. The most serious complication, frequently mentioned in the literature, is an *injury to the popliteal artery*, which, in some cases, has made a below-knee amputation necessary. A sharp, pointed knife can easily slip and penetrate the posterior capsule when the posterior horn is detached. The use of a meniscotome with adequate guards for the cutting surface will avoid this complication.

Much more frequently a large *portion of the posterior horn* remains behind, either because the meniscus tears or because it is detached too far anteriorly (Figs. 215e, f). If the posterior horn stump cannot be removed through the anterior incision without causing damage to the articular cartilage, a small incision should be made posterior to the collateral ligament, as described earlier (Figs. 212 and 213). A curved clamp or hemostat is inserted through the joint and pushed against the capsule posterior to the collateral ligament. It is then cut down upon through the second incision and the capsule is opened. This second incision is also advantageous for removal of a posterior horn left behind in a previous arthrotomy. It can also be used for removal of loose bodies from the posterior joint space.

The incision over the anterior joint space can also be used for resection of a *meniscus ganglion*. The extent of the cystic changes and accompanying damage to the meniscus can usually be evaluated from this incision. A small ganglion and the meniscus from which it arose can be detached from the capsule without much difficulty. It is obvious that in these cases the entire meniscus with its peripheral zone, from which the cystic degeneration usually arises, must be removed. If the cystic changes involve the joint capsule the skin is retracted and a second incision is made into the capsule posteriorly, over the bulge of the ganglion. It is occasionally necessary to resect a portion of the capsule with the

ganglion. Larger cysts, which present over the posterior joint space and towards the popliteal fossa, should be approached through a posterior incision. These cysts quite frequently arise from the capsule or represent a bursa. A discussion of additional operative procedures which are sometimes necessary in connection with meniscectomy, such as repair of a collateral or cruciate ligament, is outside the scope of this book. When definite meniscus pathology is present, we do not resect the infrapatellar fat pad even if some of its villi should be enlarged or fibrosed. These changes are usually secondary and resection could complicate the postoperative course unnecessarily.

After resection of the meniscus, the *wound is closed in layers*. For closure of the joint capsule we prefer to use catgut because nonabsorbable material, such as silk, cotton, etc., can occasionally lead to painful scars or stitch abscesses. The amount of suture material inside the joint cavity, however, should be kept to a minimum. Our capsular stitches do not include the synovium and the sutures are thus extra-articular. When closing the subcutaneous tissue, care must be taken not to damage the branches of the saphenous nerve. The skin is closed with interrupted silk sutures and the knee immobilized in a tight compression bandage of cotton and elastic bandages before the tourniquet is released. Postoperatively the leg is elevated in a foam rubber or basket splint in slight flexion. The skin sutures are removed on the 8th or 9th postoperative day.

### h) After-Care

The postoperative course and ultimate recovery depends to a great extent on a carefully controlled after-care. Since the condition of an operated knee joint varies from one case to another, we must avoid a rigid scheme and make the after-care as individual as possible. Two factors are important for an uneventful postoperative course:

1) Prevention of postoperative knee effusion;
2) Maintenance and/or restitution of adequate quadriceps strength.

Careful operative technic and postoperative *immobilization* are the most important measures to avoid troublesome postoperative irritation of the joint. Any traumatized tissue initially needs rest for an uneventful recovery followed by careful functional training. Proponents of systematic early mobilization who permit their patients to be up or bear weight on the second or third postoperative day after meniscectomy will experience a somewhat higher percentage of poor results.

We prefer to immobilize the knee joint on a splint during the first 3 postoperative days. After 3 days the leg is positioned on pillows and the patient is started on gentle, active motion which should not cause pain. The bandage is changed on the 8th or 9th day and the skin sutures removed. Subsequent rehabilitation depends on the condition of the knee joint. A slight effusion will develop after any articular procedure. In most cases this effusion will be completely absorbed after 8 to 10 days. The patient is then permitted to proceed with active flexion and extension exercises and is allowed out of bed as soon as he can flex the knee to a right angle. Discharge from the hospital in most cases is between the 10th and the 12th postoperative day.

If a significant effusion persists after 8 days, we prefer to aspirate the fluid, apply a compression dressing, and immobilize the knee for another 2 to 3 days. It is not advisable to discharge the patient from the hospital as long as significant irritation of the knee joint persists.

We have already mentioned that function of the quadriceps is an important factor for adequate function and stability of the knee joint. Atrophy of the vastus medialis is part of the clinical picture of any long-standing meniscus lesion. In the presence of painful limitation of extension, it is rarely possible to strengthen this muscle through exercises. Postoperative immobilization will increase muscle atrophy considerably within a few days. It is important to treat this muscle atrophy by early and systematic *active quadriceps training*. Massage, heat and other passive measures cannot replace systematic quadriceps training and we have abandoned these measures completely. The patient must be made to understand the importance of the quadriceps musculature for function of the knee joint to insure his active cooperation. Circumferential measurements of the quadriceps at regular inter-

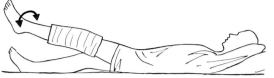

Fig. 216. Quadriceps exercises with straight leg.

vals will permit good evaluation of the patient's progress.

Quadriceps exercises should be supervised by the surgeon and should never be left to the discretion of the patient. They should be increased systematically and should be adapted to the functional condition of the knee joint. During the patient's hospitalization, quadriceps exercises should be supervised by a physiotherapist.

Muscle training is usually started on the 2nd or 3rd postoperative day. To avoid pain and irritation the patient is asked to do only isometric contractions with the knee in extension. After the third postoperative day the patient begins to do straight leg raising and to perform small circular motions with the extended leg (Fig. 216). In the beginning some assistance may be necessary but usually the resistance can be increased after a few days by addition of a small sandbag. The patient should perform this exercise for 5 minutes every hour.

As soon as the patient is able to flex his knee to a right angle – usually after the 8th to 10th day – he is asked to do extension exercises in a sitting position (Fig. 217). The patient sits on the edge of the bed or on a low table with his thigh supported by a small pillow. The knee is extended slowly but completely, held for a short period of time, and then flexed slowly. It is important that the patient use a maximum of strength and include the gluteal muscles in the exercise. The musculature should be completely relaxed between contractions. To insure good metabolic activity of the musculature, rest periods between exercises should be adequate. Occasionally it is advantageous to ask the patient to do the exercise with his normal leg first before he is asked to exercise his operated leg. As muscle function returns, resistance can be increased by loading the leg. This can be done very easily by attaching small sandbags or leg weights to the foot.

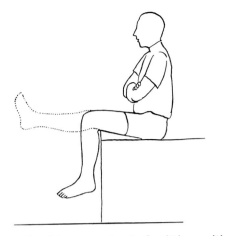

Fig. 217. Quadriceps exercises in the sitting position.

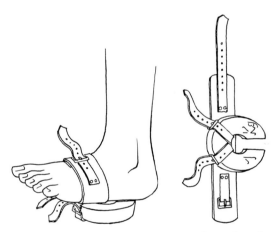

Fig. 218. Simple method to fasten weight to the sole
of the foot (modified from Smillie).

Ordinary traction weights can be used for this purpose (Fig. 218). Overexercising should be avoided. It is advisable to begin with a load of one kilogram. A load of four kilograms should not be exceeded in the beginning. If the knee shows signs of irritation or effusion, the weight must be reduced or exercises limited to the extended knee. After discharge from the hospital quadriceps exercises must be continued systematically, preferably supplemented by general conditioning exercises. It usually takes 6 to 12 weeks before normal muscle function is regained.

## 4) Postoperative Complications

### a) Postoperative Pain

Discomfort after a carefully done meniscectomy is usually minor and disappears almost completely within the first 24 hours. When quadriceps exercises are begun, muscle pull on the capsule may occasionally produce some temporary localized pain. Persistent, marked pain is usually an indication of local disturbance and must be evaluated. Usually this is due to reactive swelling after release of the tourniquet, which will disappear after further elevation of the operated leg. If this measure remains unsuccessful, the compression bandage must be loosened. Occasionally too tight a compression bandage may cause the discomfort. Marked effusion can be due to excess synovial fluid produced by the irritated synovial membrane, but much more frequently it is due to postoperative bleeding. Reaction to a bloody joint effusion varies with the individual patient. Some patients show inflammatory signs and fever, and a beginning infection cannot be ruled out. If the bloody effusion is not evacuated early enough, capsular infiltrations, adhesions, and limitation of motion may occur. After evacuation of the effusion, a new compression bandage should be applied and the joint immobilized for a few more days.

### b) Infection

The most serious complication of any arthrotomy is, without doubt, infection of the operated joint. This complication fortunately has become very rare in recent years. We have not seen an infection in our own series in the past several years even though we do not use antibiotic coverage routinely in the postoperative period.

Postoperative infections are practically always due to errors in aseptic technic. Hematogenous infections due to an undiagnosed or untreated focus of infection, such as chronic tonsillitis, dental granuloma, furuncle, or panaritium, are extremely rare. Swelling of the joint with pain, increased skin temperature and fever should always make one suspicious of infection and the necessary diagnostic and therapeutic measures must be instituted immediately. The joint must be aspirated and the fluid sent for bacteriologic examination and antibiotic sensitivity. If the aspirated fluid is cloudy we immediately begin treatment with local instillation and general administration of a broad spectrum antibiotic. The knee joint is immobilized by means of a plaster cast which is windowed over the knee. Application of traction to relieve pressure from the articular surfaces, as is frequently recommended in the literature, is of little use in the initial stage. After determination of antibiotic sensitivity we change to the most effective antibiotic. Treatment with daily joint aspirations and antibiotic instillations in combination with systematic antibiotic treatment should control most infections within a short period of time. In severe cases continued lavage of the joint should be instituted. Two thin polyethylene catheters with multiple perforations are introduced into the joint at two different locations by means of a trocar. One of the catheters is connected to a container with antibiotic solution, the other to a suction apparatus. This continued drainage of the joint can, if necessary, be carried out over several weeks, and replaces open joint drainage which very frequently leads to a stiff joint. Continuous joint lavage was used by us recently in a patient with a severely contaminated and infected knee injury. Normal range of motion was obtained even though it took approximately 6 weeks before infection subsided.

## c) Disturbances of Wound Healing

Occasionally patients will complain of considerable pain in the operative area in the first few postoperative days. Inspection will usually reveal circumscribed swelling and tension of the skin as a result of subcutaneous or intracapsular *hematomata*. These hematomas can be very annoying when they lead to adhesions between the skin and joint capsule, and produce prolonged complaints. In some cases excision of the scar may become necessary. A markedly painful hematoma should therefore be evacuated by separation of the wound or by aspiration when liquified.

Occasionally one sees a *subcutaneous seroma*. This is usually due to too loose a capsular closure that permits the synovial fluid to escape into the subcutaneous tissue. This complication can be taken care of without difficulty by aspiration of the effusion and a compression bandage.

When non-absorbable suture material is used for closure of the capsule, we occasionally see the formation of a *suture granuloma* or a *suture abscess*. These can also lead to prolonged pain and may necessitate excision of the scar. In our experience these complications usually occur in long incisions extending far beyond the femoral condyles and are not limited to the parapatellar area. Knee flexion will then stretch the scar over the femoral condyles and cause irritation. Excision of a few suture granulomata is not adequate in these cases because the complaints are due to a generalized insufficiency of the scar.

Occasionally we may encounter *neuroma* formation postoperatively from section of the infrapatellar branch of the saphenous nerve. Injuries to this nerve are not infrequent with incisions on the medial side of the knee joint. They result in anesthesia of the skin in the area of the tibial tuberosity. Vicarious innervation from the periphery will usually reduce the size of the anesthetic area over a period of several months and may eventually cause it to disappear completely.

We have no explanation why this painful neuroma develops in some patients and not in others after section of the nerve. In the hand, some authors speak of a neuroma disease. We believe that psychic factors play a significant role besides the local conditions of the scar. When the knee is moved the cut end of the nerve which is caught in the scar is pressed against the rigid surface of the tibial plateau.

Therapeutically local injections of alcohol or a depot anesthetic are of little value. The method of choice is resection of the nerve ends and suture of the nerve. After restoration of nerve function, no new neuroma will form. However, conditions for a successful secondary suture of this small nerve branch are very rarely favorable. We usually resect the proximal stump of the nerve far enough that it comes to lie in healthy well padded tissue and is no longer subjected to traction from the scar.

### d) Quadriceps Weakness

We have found that most postoperative complaints arise from inadequate strength and function of the thigh musculature. Symptomatology of quadriceps weakness is manifold. Complaints of instability, a feeling of weakness and easy fatigability predominate. Excessive use of the knee frequently causes vague pain and capsular infiltrations, occasionally even joint effusions. These symptoms usually disappear within a short time. A characteristic symptom is the so-called "giving way" which has been described previously. This occurs most frequently when walking downstairs, with sudden change of direction, or other uncontrolled motions. This sudden giving way of the knee joint which the patients frequently describe as something going out of place usually means that the vastus medialis is weak, reacts slowly, and stabilizes the knee inadequately.

These symptoms are often attributed to an error in operative technic, such as leaving the posterior horn behind or overlooking a lesion of the opposite meniscus. We have frequently seen patients who had their knee operated on a second time because of these complaints. The second operation usually does not correct the problem but quite frequently increases the quadriceps weakness. The only successful treatment in these cases is systematic and prolonged quadriceps training. It is advisable to have the patients continue their quadriceps training under the supervision of a therapist because they are usually individuals who lack the necessary drive and energy for active participation in the after-treatment.

### e) Meniscus Remnants

Occasionally the above-mentioned complaints can be due to irritation or locking from a meniscus remnant left behind at operation. We have mentioned previously that tears and detachments in the area of the posterior horn can easily be overlooked when a partial meniscectomy is carried out. Even experienced surgeons can occasionally leave a small posterior horn which later causes difficulties. It is also possible that an originally intact posterior horn remnant can tear and cause locking.

The patient's complaints from this condition, like those from quadriceps weakness, are not very characteristic. Localized tenderness over the posterior joint space is rarely present. The patients complain of vague discomfort in the joint and a feeling of instability or "giving way" when they walk. Occasionally they describe snapping sounds or slight catching which usually occurs with rotary motions or when coming up from a squatting position.

When these complaints persist despite intensive quadriceps training, we usually examine the knee by arthrography. We have found arthrography to be a valuable diagnostic tool to clarify postoperative complaints. It has helped us reduce the number of reoperations considerably. Arthrographic findings, on the other hand, have frequently convinced us that reoperation is necessary as shown in the following case:

B. C., 37-year-old male office worker. Medial meniscectomy of the left knee on 2/10/1954 with removal of a torn degenerated meniscus (preoperative arthrography was not done because of clear-cut symptomatology). Following return to work, the patient soon developed locking episodes. A lesion of the lateral meniscus was suspected but arthrography revealed a torn posterior horn remnant (Fig. 154). Re-arthrotomy confirmed this and the patient has remained asymptomatic.

### f) Chronic Synovitis

Occasionally irritation of the joint with capsular infiltration and effusion can develop postoperatively and lead to permanent joint disability. This can be due to a variety of causes which have already been discussed in previous chapters. The following is a brief summary of the different causes of chronic synovitis:

a) *Surgical trauma* (prolonged operation, difficult meniscectomy with considerable trauma to joint capsule and articular cartilage);

b) *Postoperative hemarthrosis;*

c) *Quadriceps weakness* (instability of the knee joint, recurrent subluxations);

d) *Excessive stress* (weight bearing too early, forced quadriceps training, etc.);

e) *Pre-existing joint damage* (local cartilaginous lesions from long-standing meniscus tears, generalized arthrosis, ligamentous damage, unstable knee);

g) *Infectious arthritis* (focal infections from chronic tonsillitis, dental granulomata, etc.).

When the cause of chronic postoperative synovitis has been established, the proper *treatment* can be instituted in most cases. Quite frequently it is sufficient to reduce the patient's activity and limit his quadriceps training to isometric exercises with the knee extended. Moist warm packs will considerably influence resorption of a persistent capsular infiltration. If effusion recurs rapidly after aspiration, intra-articular injection of hydrocortisone can be tried. Joint infection must be ruled out first since intra-articular cortisone injection in the presence of a joint infection can lead to catastrophic results. In severe cases, prolonged complete immobilization with bed rest or a plaster cast may be necessary. Windowing the capsule and total synovectomy have been suggested for treatment of chronic joint effusions. Thus far we have never found it necessary to resort to one of these methods.

The following case illustrates some of the difficulties which can arise occasionally:

A. B.: A 32-year-old merchant sustained a contusion of the medial side of the right knee in August of 1958 when he hit it with a hatchet. This resulted in a joint effusion of short duration. Because of persistent complaints the intact medial meniscus was excised elsewhere in January of 1959. The patient was permitted out of bed on the 3rd postoperative day and was discharged on the 7th day. Joint effusion developed again and persisted despite prolonged bandaging and treatment with diathermy, hot packs, etc. Cultures of the joint fluid for tuberculosis were negative. A pneumo-arthrogram in August of 1959 did not show any abnormal findings. Ten X-ray treatments of the knee joint did not give any relief. Examination of tonsils and teeth did not reveal any pathology. Despite his difficulties the patient never lost a day of work. After the effusion had persisted for more than a year, the patient was admitted to our hospital in February of 1960. The right knee joint revealed considerable effusion and diffuse thickening of the capsule. Marked quadriceps atrophy was present. One hundred cc. of clear yellow effusion was aspirated. Bacteriologic examination was negative. The patient was placed on strict bed rest, low salt diet and a diuretic. The leg was immobilized on a splint for 10 days, followed by isometric quadriceps exercises. A 2-week course of prednisone was given in addition to intra-articular cortisone injections every 3 days. Local treatment consisted of daily moist compresses. With this treatment the effusions regressed slowly and had disappeared completely after 5 weeks. Some infiltration of the capsule persisted. The patient was discharged with a cylinder cast after 6 weeks. Isometric quadriceps training was continued by the patient at home. The cylinder cast was removed after 4 weeks and the knee joint appeared to be asymptomatic. During the following weeks mild effusions recurred after excessive use but always disappeared overnight. The patient is completely asymptomatic since the fall of 1960 and can carry on his usual activities, including tennis and skiing, without limitations.

## g) Sudeck's Dystrophy

Sudecks dystrophy occasionally develops after injuries, infections, or operative procedures on the lower leg or the hand but can also occur in the area of the knee joint. The symptoms in the knee region are usually less pronounced than those in the more peripheral areas.

We should always suspect a Sudeck's dystrophy when the patients complain of persistent vague *pain* after a meniscus operation and we are unable to find any cause for it. Pain and soft tissue changes are the main symptoms in the beginning. The joint capsule and subcutaneous tissue are edematous initially. Later they become hard and infiltrated. Skin temperature is markedly elevated, the skin is tight and occasionally reddened. Knee flexion is characteristically limited and painful from the beginning. After a few weeks edema and inflammatory changes decrease and are replaced by a diffuse induration of the capsule. Patients complain of swelling and pain after increased activity for many months. These symptoms are localized mainly in the suprapatellar pouch and in the parapatellar region. Typical bony changes of spotty osteoporosis are usually not visible before 6 or 8 weeks and are primarily seen in the patella (Fig. 219). Demineralization of the femoral condyles is seen less frequently.

A diagnosis of Sudeck's dystrophy is important to determine the choice of treatment and for the prognosis. It is important for both the surgeon and the patient to realize that disability will be prolonged.

All measures which produce pain and irritation of tissues must be avoided. In the initial stage sedation with tranquilizers plus a 2-week course of cortisone, with high oral doses for the

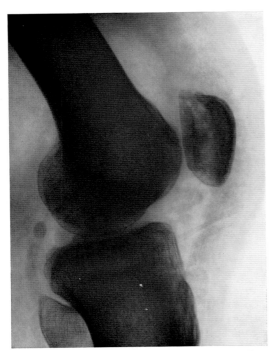

Fig. 219. Sudeck's dystrophy. Predominant involvement of the patella.

first week and decreasing doses during the second week, are frequently of benefit.

After the acute phase has subsided, careful physical therapy with Hauffe baths, connective tissue massage and carefully increasing isometric exercises should be started. Passive exercises and joint manipulation should be avoided because they frequently cause an acute flare-up of the Sudeck's syndrome. Anabolic steroids and intraarticular cortisone injections are frequently of benefit. We also recommend treatment with sympathetic blocks. Early and repeated blocks of the lumbar sympathetic chain will in many cases cause rapid regression of pain and soft tissue infiltrations. Psychological treatment must also be included in the therapy of Sudeck's dystrophy because endogenous psychic factors are probably involved in the development of this syndrome.

## h) Arthrosis Deformans

A discussion of arthrosis deformans should be included in the chapter of postoperative complications. After the age of 40 and especially after a long-standing meniscus lesion, we regularly find degenerative changes of the joint surfaces. The trauma of surgery can frequently cause a flare-up of arthrotic symptoms. The symptomatology of arthrosis deformans has already been discussed in the chapter on differential diagnosis. The signs and symptoms of chronic synovitis usually predominate.

Treatment consists of all forms of physical therapy such as baths and heat applications, which can be augmented by cortisone or X-ray treatment.

Arthrosis deformans can influence the long-term prognosis after meniscus operations considerably. In Schaer's series the 10-year results were good and excellent in 80 per cent of the cases. This is approximately what can be expected today because quite often irreversible changes are present preoperatively. We feel, however, that the long-term results after meniscus damage are influenced considerably by medical and surgical measures. Our results will be best if we apply the age-old principle of "primum nil nocere." The operation should be performed only when it is definitely indicated, with careful handling of the tissues and with adequate aftercare.

# CHAPTER 8

# Disability Evaluation

The majority of our population is insured against injuries and disease. This means that in most meniscus lesions the question of the cause may have to be evaluated. All insurance carriers, whether governmental, industrial, or private, have certain regulations for coverage which from time to time are adapted to the newest medical standards. These regulations differ considerably from one state to another. The literature also shows a considerable discrepancy of opinions. The following is a discussion of some of the basic questions which may facilitate the evaluation of these lesions.

In the chapter on the pathogenesis of meniscus lesions we have already discussed that we are dealing with two main factors in the etiology of these lesions. The role which each of these factors play must be carefully evaluated for each meniscus damage. The two factors are traumatic *meniscus injury* and gradual degeneration of the meniscus on the basis of increased stress *(meniscopathy)* which can lead to spontaneous detachment of the meniscus.

The importance of *primary degeneration* has been overrated considerably. Physiologically we are able to find degenerative changes of the menisci in almost all people after the third decade. These changes do not alter the tensile strength of the cartilages significantly. If this physiologic degeneration were of any significance, the incidence of meniscus lesions should increase with advancing age. This, however, is not the case. We can show statistically that without any doubt the majority of meniscus lesions falls in the 3rd and 4th decades. This is the age group where the knee joints are exposed quite frequently to sports and industrial injuries. Another argument against the importance of physiologic degeneration and constitutional inferiority is the fact that meniscus injuries are much more frequent in men than in women. Meyer has shown recently, on the basis of private insurance company statistics, that wo-

men with their increasing participation in sports now submit as many claims for meniscus lesions as men. Prolonged mechanical stress, like that produced by work in a kneeling position, such as in mining, floor laying, stonecutting, gardening, cleaning, etc., is necessary to produce pathologic changes which reduce the tensile strength of the meniscus significantly. This prolonged work in a kneeling position causes pressure damage of the menisci between the articular surfaces. Ground substance and fibers degenerate and become necrotic. The meniscus becomes more vulnerable and can tear spontaneously without external trauma. The clinical picture is frequently not very characteristic. The knee joint does not show any signs of acute trauma, but limitation of motion is obvious. At operation the menisci usually show extensive degenerative changes both macroscopically and microscopically, combined with circumscribed connective tissue scarring. The surface of the meniscus shows yellow discoloration and considerable fraying. One or more longitudinal tears are usually present in the avascular inner zone of the menisci. The lesion predominantly involves the medial meniscus and is frequently bilateral.

The Bochum clinic (Magnus, Andreesen, and Buerkle de la Camp) deserves credit for clarifying the importance of meniscopathy in miners which has led to its recognition as an industrial disease. Meniscus lesions in miners are now recognized as industrial disabilities after the patient has worked regularly as a miner for a period of 3 years. It is quite possible that in the future this ruling will be extended to other vocations which require prolonged work in a kneeling position. Swiss industrial insurance does not cover meniscopathy as an industrial disability. These cases can, however, be accepted as industrial disability on an individual basis.

With the exception of mining areas the percentage of spontaneous detachments in the total number of meniscus lesions is relatively small. According to the statistical analyses of Bossard, Fehr, and Groh, they make up only 2 to 4 per cent of the total.

In the majority of cases a meniscus lesion is the *result of an injury*. Magnus and also Buerkle de la Camp recommend that a meniscus lesion should be recognized as an industrial disability only in those cases where adequate external trauma has injured the knee and resulted in limitation of motion of the knee joint, formation of an effusion and inability to bear weight on the leg, causing the patient to stop working immediately.

Böhler does not agree with this opinion. He maintains that the conditions mentioned above are rarely the cause of an industrial meniscus lesion. In his opinion, the trauma is usually indirect, not direct. It does not require great force to produce the lesion. A quick turning motion with the knee in slight flexion represents adequate trauma. Pain is usually not very severe and the patient often does not stop working. The pain becomes more severe with locking. Effusion is often minimal and usually not bloody. Breitenfelder maintains that a bloody effusion is always caused by an injury to capsule or bone.

Meyer goes even further and recommends that all meniscus injuries which cause locking and are proven at surgery, even those without adequate trauma, should be accepted by the insurance company if the patient has been insured with them for a minimum of 2 years.

We agree with Böhler, Breitenfelder, Groh, Kroemer and others, that the above-mentioned criteria of Magnus do not apply in most cases. Our position is based mainly on the following two arguments:

1) We have already mentioned that a meniscus injury is sustained most frequently from indirect trauma and rarely from a direct trauma. Due to their long levers, the muscles within the body can develop enough force to tear a normal meniscus even without a major external force (Kallius, Groh). The decisive factor, in our opinion, is not the extent of the external force but a sudden disturbance in the normal function of the knee joint. Forces sufficient to tear a healthy meniscus can arise from a combination of rotation with flexion-extension motions in the knee joint. A sudden twisting motion of the body can trap the meniscus between the bony condyles of the tibia and femur and cause a crushing or tearing injury. This explains why a meniscus can be torn even when the injury appears to be insignificant.

2) The opinion that all meniscus injuries produce marked clinical symptoms can no longer be upheld today. We know from experience that total longitudinal tears which lead to immediate blocking of the knee joint do not usually occur with the first injury to a healthy meniscus. Much more frequently, the first injury results in partial detachment from the joint capsule or a partial tear in the cartilaginous substance. If this injury is limited to the avascular nerve-free inner zone of the meniscus, the symptoms will be minimal and only a mild-to-moderate serous effusion develops. When symptoms are minimal the patient does not always stop working to consult a doctor. If the meniscus lesion is close to the capsule, it can heal or quiet down sufficiently so that the patient becomes asymptomatic for many weeks, months, or even years without any disability. When the primary injury does not heal adequately, further stress on the knee will, sooner or later, lead to new symptoms and gradual extension of the original tear even without a new injury. This can then lead to sudden locking of the knee without significant trauma.

Krömer distinguishes between meniscus lesions resulting from one injury and meniscus lesions which result from multiple traumatic episodes. This concept is confusing because the first injury is the important one as far as recognition of the lesion by the insurance company is concerned. Any subsequent disturbance is a result of this original injury.

A *traumatic tear* subsequently leads to secondary degenerative changes which frequently are difficult to distinguish from primary degeneration of the meniscus, even as soon as 6 to 8 weeks after the original injury. For many years insurance companies have placed considerable emphasis on histopathologic findings in the excised meniscus. This position has been weakened considerably in the last few years. As early as 1946 Lang insisted that histology should play only a secondary role in disability evaluation of a meniscus lesion.

When the meniscus lesion occurs as a late change in an unstable knee after ligamentous injury, its evaluation is usually not too difficult. If the original ligamentous lesion is covered by insurance, the insurance company is also responsible for the secondary meniscus lesion.

Evaluation of a meniscus lesion should always be based on thorough consideration of all factors, including history, mechanisms of injury, as well as clinical, X-ray, operative and histologic findings. In many cases, the traumatic origin of the lesion cannot be established with certainty and we have to be satisfied with a probability.

When taking the *history,* it is important to ask about duration of symptoms. A fresh injury with typical trauma usually does not pose any difficulty and the insurance company will usually accept the claim. Much more frequently we find that the complaints have been present for some time. In these cases it is important to find the cause for the initial symptoms. This original injury may have occured months and years earlier, but must have been adequate to injure a healthy meniscus. The patient's intermittent symptoms may have been only minimal, such as mild discomfort in the knee with certain activities. Occasional sudden "giving way" of the knee or a painful snap in the knee are very characteristic symptoms.

Occasionally the patient does not remember an earlier injury. It is then important to find out about previous *sports* activities such as soccer, skiing, track and field, wrestling, or skating. Thorough interrogation of the patient will frequently reveal a previous injury to the knee which at the time was diagnosed and treated as a sprain and which the patient does not connect with his present condition.

Another important factor is the patient's present or previous *vocational* activity, which may have caused premature degeneration of his menisci. In order to have a meniscopathy recognized as an industrial disability, it must be shown that the patient has done work in a kneeling position for many years. The simple fact that the patient has worked underground is usually not sufficient. He must be able to show that he

has actually mined coal in low mine shafts in a kneeling position for several years (Andreesen). Exact reconstruction of the original injury is frequently impossible or, at best, very difficult. The trauma to the knee is frequently indirect and occurs in a matter of seconds. The patient's own history of the injury is often vague and not very accurate. Thorough interrogation of the patient will occasionally clarify the mechanism of injury, but in many cases we must be satisfied to settle for the most probable cause.

Traumatic episodes which can cause damage to a meniscus are manifold. The most frequent mechanism is a forceful rotatory stress on the knee as it occurs with sudden torsion of the body when the foot is fixed, or a sudden slipping of the foot when the thigh is fixed. A fall, stumbling, a missed step, or a sudden evasive motion are all mechanisms which can injure a meniscus. The characteristic denominator in all these episodes is the sudden twisting force which acts on the usually flexed knee joint.

A *joint effusion* is probably the most consistent *clinical finding* following an injury to the knee. A bloody effusion is usually indicative of a traumatic meniscus lesion, especially when there are signs and symptoms of damage to capsule and ligamentous structures. Spontaneous detachment of the meniscus very rarely causes bleeding into the joint, but it can occur occasionally after spontaneous detachment close to the capsule. Many fresh meniscus injuries produce only a serous effusion.

The amount and nature of the joint effusion do not permit any conclusions as to the etiology of the meniscus lesion, nor does the degree of pain, the limitation of motion, and the inability to bear weight. The immediate symptoms after a total spontaneous detachment of the meniscus can be more severe than those of an incomplete fresh traumatic rupture.

The condition of the patient's *musculature* and the X-ray occasionally give us valuable information about a pre-existing lesion of the meniscus. When considerable quadriceps atrophy is present immediately after the injury, we can assume that the leg has been favored for quite some time. Localized arthrotic changes on the X-ray, especially a bony ridge on the tibial plateau, usually indicate that damage to the meniscus has been present for many months or years.

*Operative findings and histological examination* can be used for clarification of the etiology of the meniscus lesion only in those cases where surgery was performed shortly after the injury in question. A bloody or xanthochrome effusion, bloody imbibition in the area of the tear or the adjacent joint capsule, a sharply delineated, ragged tear, and a shiny grayish white surface of the meniscus are usually indicative of a fresh injury. If subsequent histologic examination does not show any significant degenerative changes, we must assume that this meniscus lesion was caused by the injury in question, even in those cases where the trauma was not very significant.

Only a few weeks after the initial injury the edges of the tear begin to smooth off and secondary degenerative changes develop in the area of the tear, especially in the detached frag-ment. These secondary degenerative changes are frequently indistinguishable from those of primary meniscus degeneration. The microscopic findings in late cases can be used in favor of a traumatic etiology of the meniscus lesion only when the degenerative changes are limited to the area of the tear and the remainder of the cartilage appears healthy. The presence of degenerative changes in late cases, on the other hand, does not necessarily indicate a pathologic meniscopathy without any connection to the injury in question. Only thorough examination and evaluation of all factors, including history and physical findings, will permit a valid conclusion.

In borderline cases we usually assume a traumatic origin of the lesion since statistically injuries play a much greater role in the etiology of meniscus lesions than does abnormal primary degeneration.

# Bibliography

AARSTRAND, T.: Treatment of meniscal rupture of the knee joint. A follow-up examination of material where only the ruptured part of the meniscus has been removed. Acta chir. scand. (Stockh.) 107 (1954), 146

AMORTH, G., T. PASQUINELLI: Artrografia con mezzo di contrasto idrosolubile e sua utilità nella diagnosis delle lesioni meniscali. Scritti in onore di R. Balli, Coop. Tip., Modena (1955)

ANDERSEN, K.: Pneumoarthrography of the knee joint with particular reference to the semilunar cartilages. Acta orthop. scand. Suppl. 4 (1948)
Some experience with a new method for arthrography. Acta Radiol. 25 (1944), 33

ANDREESEN, R.: Meniskusbeschädigungen (Verletzungen und Erkrankungen bei Sport und Arbeit). Erg. Chir. 30 (1937), 24
Schienbeinkopfbrüche und ihre Behandlung. Vortr. prakt. Chir. H. 91, F. Enke, Stuttgart 1955
Meniskusschäden bei Bergleuten. In: Handbuch der gesamten Arbeitsmedizin. Urban & Schwarzenberg, Munich and Berlin 1961
Geschichtliche Entwicklung und Grundlagen der Berufskrankheit 42 (Bergmanns-Meniscus). Z. Unfallheilk. 66 (1963) 196

ANDRÉN, L., L. WEHLIN: Double-contrast arthrography of knee with horizontal roentgen-ray beam. Acta orthop. scand. 29 (1960), 307

ANTOINE, M., J. LESURE, J. CREUSOT: L'arthrographie du genou par contraste opaque. J. Radiol. Électrol. 36 (1955), 215

ANZILOTTI, A.: Tumore primitivo della sinoviale articolare. Communicazione al XVIII Congr. Soc. Ital. di Ortopedia, Bologna 1927

APLEY, A. C.: The diagnosis of meniscal injuries. J. Bone Jt. Surg. 29 (1947), 78

ARCHIMBAUD, J.: Diagnostic des lésions méniscales et ligamentaires du genou par l'arthrographie. Thèse Lyon 1950
Quelques problèmes particuliers concernant la pneumoarthrographie du genou. Memoires, Lyons 1951

ARENS, A., M. BERNSTEIN: Diagnostic inflation of the knee joint. A clinical radiological study. Radiology, 7 (1926), 500

ATTILJ, S.: L'indagine radiologica delle lesioni meniscali del ginocchio. Stud. med. chir. sport. 2 (1948), 47

BALENSWEIG, J., G. IRVING: Loose body in knee joint demonstrated by pneumoarthrosis. Surg. Gynec. Obstet. 39, (1934), 235

BARUCHA, E.: Wschr. Unfallheilk. 63 (1960), 370

BASSET, J.: Le genou. Masson, Paris 1932

BAUMGARTL, F., A. DAHM: Zur Pathogenese der Osteochondritis dissecans. Zbl. Chir. 87 (1942), 1916

BEAU, H., P. L. GÉRARD: Valeur comparative des diverses tecniques d'arthrographie du genou. J. Radiol. Électrol. 36 (1955), 467

BECKER, F.: Neuläsion eines echten Meniskusregenerates. Helv. med. Acta 3 (1936), 871
Zerreißung eines echten Meniskusregenerates. Chirurg 8 (1936), 680

BERG, R. F.: An improved air injection apparatus for the inflation of joints. Amer. J. Surg. 8 (1930), 1277

BESSLER, W., A. RÜTTIMANN: Die Röntgensymptome der Synovitis villosa des Kniegelenkes. Fortschr. Röntgenstr. 99 (1963), 343

BESTLE, S.: Meniskusschaden und Sport. Med. Klin. 50 (1955), 283

BETTINELLI, G., G. L. PALEARI: La nostra esperienza sull'artrografia del ginocchio. Arch. Ortop. (Milan) 73 (1960), 992
–, G. L. PALEARI: Esperienza personale con l'artrografia del ginocchio. Arch. Ortop. (Milan) 73 (1960), 992

BIONDETTI, P.: Artrografia opaca del ginocchio. Minerva med. 50 (1959), 3611
Quadri artrografici del ginocchio. Comunicaz. XXXVI Raduno Triveneto, Rovigo 15–11, 1958; Radiol. med. (Turin) 45 (1959), 71

BIRCHER, E., J. OBERHOLZER: Die Kniegelenkkapsel im Pneumoradiographiebild Acta. radiol. 15 (1934), 452
Die Binnenverletzungen des Kniegelenkes. Schweiz. med. Wschr. 59 (1929), 1292; 1309

BLONEK, F., J. WOLF: Pneumoradiography of the knee joint. J. Iowa St. Med. Soc. 34 (1944), 354

BLUMENSAAT, C.: Meniscusregenerat und Berufskrankheit No. 26. Mschr. Unfallheilk. 61 (1958), 33

BOBBIO, A., A. PICCO: Ricerche sperimentali sullo studio delle articolazioni mediante introduzione di liquidi opachi. Arch. ital. Chir. 34 (1933), 2

BÖHLER, L.: Behandlungsergebnisse der operierten Meniskusverletzungen. Wien. klin. Wschr. 05 (1938), 1166
Behandlung, Nachbehandlung und Begutachtung von Meniskusverletzungen. Erfahrungen an 1000 operierten Fällen. Langenbecks Arch. klin. Chir. 282 (1955), 264
Die Technik der Knochenbruchbehandlung, 12/13 ed. Vol. II, Part 2, W. Maudrich, Vienna 1957

BÖHLER, J.: Zur Pneumoarthrographie des Kniegelenkes. Amer. J. Med., 65 (1951), 398

BÖHM, M.: Die Darstellung des Gelenkknorpels im Röntgenbild. Fortschr. Röntgenstr. 44 (1931), 536

BOKSHTEIN, M. E., M. S. LEIKINA: K voprosu o kontrastnom issledovanü kolennogo sustava pri povrezhdenüakh meniskov – Ortop. traum. protez. Moskva 19 (1958), 32

BOMBELLI, R.: Sulla vascolarizzazione dei menischi umani. Arch. ortop. Milano 70 (1957), 336
Sulla vascolarizzazione dei menischi articolari del ginocchio nel coniglio. Arch. ortop. Milano 70 (1957), 119

BONNIN, I. G.: Cysts of the semilunar cartilages of the knee
–, BOLDERO: The arthrography of the knee joint. Surgery 85 (1947), 64
–, F. R. BERIDGE: The radiographic examination of the ankle joint including arthrography. Amer. J. Med. 64 (1947), 793

BOREŠ, J.: Our experience with arthrography of the knee made seriographically under skiascopic control. Čs. Rentgenol. 12 (1958), 179

BOROW, L. S.: Arthrogr. II. The evaluation of pneumoarthrographs. Brit. J. Radiol. 25 (1952), 129

BOSSARD, M.: Erfahrungen mit 500 Meniscus-Operationen bei Versicherten der Schweiz. Unfallversicherungsanstalt in den Jahren 1952/53. Diss. Zurich 1955

BOURDON, R., J. BESSON, C. MASSARE, M. DUCOUT: A propos of pneumoarthrography of the knee. The problem of protection in direct radiological examination. Gaz. méd. Fr. 67 (1960), 1107
–, J. BESSON, M. BARD, J. CEDAHA: Dispositif de pneumoarthrographie du genou. J. radiol. électr. 39 (1958), 689

BOYD, D.: Knee joint visualization: a roentgenographic study with Iopax. J. Bone J. Surg. 16 (1934), 671

BRAGARD, K.: Ein neues Meniscuszeichen. Münch. med. Wschr. 77 (1930), 682

BRAUS, H.: Anatomie des Menschen. 2nd ed. J. Springer, Berlin 1929

BREITENFELDER, H.: Die Begutachtung des Unfallzusammenhanges der Meniscusbeschädigung. Unfallheilk. H. 57, J. Springer, Berlin 1958

BROOKE, H. H. W., W. C. MACKENZIE, J. R. SMITH: Pneumoroentgenography with oxygen in diagnosis of internal derangements of the knee joint. Amer. J. Roentgenol. 54 (1945), 462

BÜCKART, K.: Kontrastdarstellung der Gelenke. Zbl. Chir. 60 (1933), 2185

BURCKHARDT, E.: Perthes. Osteochondritis dissecans und Coxa vara infantum im Tierexperiment. Helv. chir. Acta 15 (1948), 3

BURCKHARDT, H.: Über Entstehung freier Gelenkkörper und über die Mechanik des Kniegelenkes. Bruns' Beitr. klin. Chir. 130 (1923), 163

BURI, P., M. GEISER: Beitrag zum Problem der Aetiologie und Pathogenese der Osteochondritis dissecans am Kniegelenk. Z. Unfallmed. Berufskr. 55 (1962), 95

BÜRKLE DE LA CAMP, H.: Über Meniscusschäden. Arch. orthop. Chir. 3 (1936), 37
Meniskusverletzung und Meniskusschaden. Wien. med. Wschr. 107 (1957), 869
Meniskusverletzungen und Meniskusschäden. Ihre Erkennung und Behandlung. Therapiewoche 8 (1957), 106
Bänder- und Binnenschäden des Kniegelenkes. Chirurg 8 (1959), 374
-, P. ROSTOCK: Handbuch der gesamten Unfallheilkunde, 2nd ed. F. Enke, Stuttgart 1956
BURMANN, M. S., I. S. TUMIK, M. POMERANZ: The injection of lipiodol into the knee joint. A warning against its use. Amer. J. Roentgenol. 28 (1932), 787
BUTTS, J. B., J. T. MITCHELL: Pneumoroentgenarthrography as a diagnostic aid in internal derangements of the knee. U.S. nav. med. Bull. 46 (1946), 77

CABOT, J. R.: Resultados de la meniscectomia en los 800 primeros casos. Med. clin. (Barcelona) 20 (1953), 19
La neumografia en el diagnostico de los traumas meniscales de la rodilla. Med. esp. 7 (1946), 327
Traumatologia de los meniscos de la rodilla. Editorial Paz Montalvo, Madrid 1951
CAMLI, N.: Study of meniscal lesions of the knee using contrast arthrography. Istanbul Üniv. Tip. Fak. Mec. 22 (1959), 358
CANDARDJIS, G., F. SAEGESSER: L'arthrographie du genou par la méthode du double contraste. Radiol. Clinica, 22 (1953), 521
L'arthrographie du genou par la méthode du double contraste. Vie méd. 37 (1956).
CANIGIANI, TH., H. PIRKER: Die Kontrastfüllung des Kniegelenkes zur Diagnostik der Meniscusschäden in der Praxis. Münch. med. Wschr. 82 (1935), 1871
CARLOSTELLA, F.: La pneumoartrografia nelle lesioni traumatiche dei menischi del ginocchio. Riv. Infort. Mal. prof. 45 (1958), 465
CASTELLANA, A.: Le lesioni delle cartilagini meniscali del ginocchio (Studio Clinico statistico). Minerva ortop. 5 (1954), 97
CATTANEO, F.: Pneumartrografia diagnostica in un caso di frattura del menisco ed in un altro con lipoma arborescente del ginocchio. Boll. Special. med. chir., 3 (1929), 44
CATOLLA CAVALCANTI, G., G. FARINET: Alcune considerazioni sull'incidenza e sul trattamento fisioterapeutico delle ossificazioni paracondiloidee femorali mediali in rapporto a traumatismi gravi. Minerva fisioter. 3 (1958), 20
Ricerche artrografiche con mezzo di contrasto combinato nelle lesioni meniscali del ginocchio. Minerva fisioter. 4 (1959), 185
Diagnosi clinica e radiologica delle fratture meniscali del ginocchio. Ediz. Minvera Medica, Turin 1963
Diagnosi clinica e radiologica delle fratture meniscali del ginocchio. Ed. Minvera Medica Turin, 1963
CAVALLETTI, V., R. MEMMI: Contributo al rilievo radiografico delle lesioni dei menischi del ginocchio. Ortop. Traum. Appar. mot. 6 (1934), 163
CAVE, E. F.: Combined anterior-posterior approach to the knee joint. J. Bone Surg. 17 (1935), 427
CEELEN, W.: Über histologische Meniskusbefunde nach Unfallverletzungen. Zbl. Chir. 68 (1941), 1491
Zur Meniscus-Pathologie. Ärztl. Wschr. 8 (1953), 337
CHAPCHAL, G.: Grundsätzliche Fragen der Diagnostik und Therapie der Meniskusverletzungen. Sportärztl. Prax. 1 (1958), 17
CHAUVIN, E., Y. BOURDE: Articular pneumoserosa of the knee in the diagnosis of meniscal lesions. Rev. Orthop. 12 (1925), 137
CHILDRESS, H. M.: Popliteal cysts associated with undiagnosed posterior lesions of the medial meniscus. J. Bone Surg. 36 A (1954), 1233
Diagnosis of posterior lesions of the medial meniscus. Description of a new test. Amer. J. Surg. 93 (1957), 782
CIPRIANI, G.: Sulle lesioni dei menischi del ginocchio. Arch. Ortop. 45 (1929), 120
CIRILLO, L., E. BOSCHIN: Studio della struttura e delle caratteristiche architettoniche del menisco rigenerato. Chir. Ital. 11 (1959), 477
CLAUSEN, A.: Beitrag zur Frage positives oder negatives Kontrastmittel bei Kniegelenkarthrographien. Fortschr. Röntgenstr. 65 (1942), 76

COLANERI, L. J.: Possono essere chiarite le lesioni meniscali dal riempimento dell'articolazione mediante ossigeno? Clinique 21 (1926), 385
CONGIU, A., E. PIRASTU: Pneumostratigrafia del ginocchio. Comunic. al XVII Congr. It. di Rad. Med. Atti Vol. II, 275 (1952)
CORREA, T., A. BOTELHEIRO: A arthropneumographia no diagnostico das lesoes traumaticas dos meniscos. Gaz. Med. Portug. 1 (1948), 515
COURVOISIER, E.: Sur la régénération des ménisques du genou après méniscectomie. Helv. chir. Acta 26 (1959), 358
CROONENBERGHS, P., R. ROMBOUTS: Quelques réflexions à propos d'une centaine d'arthrographies mixtes en série du genou. Journ. Belge radiol. 36 (1953), 481
-, R. ROMBOUTS: Quelques réflexions à propos de 91 arthrographies du genou. Acta orthop. belg. 19 (1953), 307
CULLEN, C. H., G. Q. CHANGE: Air arthrography in lesions of the semilunar cartilages. Brit. J. Surg. 30 (1943), 241

D'AMORE, T.: Il valore della pneumoarthrografia nella diagnosi di lesione meniscale. Minerva ortop. 3 (1952), 27
DE PALMA, A. F.: Diseases of the Knee. Management in Medicine and Surgery. J. B. Lippincott, Philadelphia 1954
DEL BUONO, M., A. RÜTTIMANN: L'artrografia del ginocchio. Il Pensiero Scientifico Editore, Rome 1959
-, A. RÜTTIMANN: L'Artrografia del ginocchio con doppio mezzo di contrasto. Comunicaz. XXXVI Radun o Gruppo Triveneto, Rovigo 16.11.1958; Rad. med. 1 (1959), 71
DELLA SANTA, A.: Sulla visibilità dei menischi del ginocchio. Radiol. med. 22 (1935), 929
DÉTRIE, P.: La méniscectomie de Bosworth. Presse méd. 62 (1954), 1430
DIETRICH, H.: Die Regeneration des Meniscus. Dtsch. Z. Chir. 230 (1931), 251
DJIAN, A., R. CALOP, H. PUCHOT: Méniscographie du genou. Rev. prat. Par. 8 (1958), 3045
-, R. CALOP, H. PUCHOT: Chondrography of the knee. The radioclinical diagnosis of chondritis and osteochondritis. Rev. Rhum. 27 (1960), 401
-, R. CALOP, H. PUCHOT: Méniscographie en série du genou à double contraste. Atlas de radiologie clinique. Presse méd. 57 (1959), 1
DITTMAR, O.: Der Kniegelenkmeniscus im Röntgenbild. Röntgenpraxis 4 (1942), 442
DOMINGUEZ NAVARRO, L.: El diagnostico de la fractura de menisco. Rec. Esp. Cir. 3 (1946), 40
DURANTI, M.: Esempi di artrografie del ginocchio eseguite con mezzo di contrasto radiopaco (Tecnica di Lindblom). G. Med. milit. CIV (1954), 177

ECOIFFIER, J.: Arthrographie opaque. Cours de radiologie à la Clinique Médicale du Pr. Coste. France méd. 1955
Arthrographie du genou avec simple et double contraste. France méd. 18 (1955), 3
EGGELIN, W.: Zur Diagnostik der Meniskusverletzung unter Berücksichtigung der Pneumoradiographie. Zbl. Chir. 84 (1959), 241
EKBLOM, T., G. KLEFENBERG: Arthrography in the diagnosis of rupture of the quadriceps tendon. Opusc. med. (Stockh.) 1 (1956), 190
ENGELMAYER, E., U. FARKAŠ: Direktnativna meniskografia. čs. Rentgenol. 13 (1959), 153
EPSTEIN, J.: Kontrastfüllungen des Kniegelenkes mit Abrodil. Zbl. Chir. 58 (1931), 2507
EVANS, W. A.: The roentgenological demonstration of the true articular space, with particular reference to the knee joint and the internal semilunar cartilage. Amer. J. Roentgenol. 43 (1940), 860

FAIRBANK, T. J.: Knee changes after meniscectomy. J. Bone Surg. 30 (1948), 666
FEHR, A. M.: Differentialdiagnose der Kniegelenksaffektionen. Schweiz. Z. Tbk. 9 (1952), 370
FEHR, P.: Die histologische Untersuchung des verletzten Meniskus nach topographischen Gesichtspunkten. Z. Unfallmed. Berufskr. 39 (1946), 5
FERRERO, V.: Le lesion delle fibrocartilagini semilunari dell'articolazione del ginocchio. Chir. Org. Movi, X. A. 10 (1925—26), 317

FICAT, P.: Contribution à l'étude arthrographique de la gonarthrose. Diplôme d'Electroradiologie, Toulouse 1954
FISCHEDICK, O., P. SOCHA: Indikation und Ergebnisse der Kontrastdarstellung des Kniegelenkes mit positivem Kontrastmittel. Chirurg 31 (1960), 13
Erfahrungen bei der Arthrographie des Kniegelenkes mit positivem Kontrastmittel. Röntgen-Bl. 13 (1960), 337
FISCHER, A. W., G. ROLINEUS: Das ärztliche Gutachten im Versicherungswesen. J. A. Barth, Munich 1955
FISHER, A. G. T.: A new method of approach to the semilunar cartilages of the knee joint. Lancet 1931/II, 1407
Internal Derangements of the Knee Joint. H. K. Lewis, London 1933
FISCHER, F. K.: In: Schinz, Baensch, Friedl, Uehlinger, Lehrbuch der Röntgendiagnostik. 5th ed. G. Thieme, Stuttgart 1951
FONTAINE, R., R. RABER, P. WARTER, W. MONTORSI, J. N. MÜLLER: L'arthropneumographie du genou. Technique et résultats dans 50 affections méniscales. Rev. chir. 71 (1952), 327
FORSTER, E., L. MOLÉ, R. PETER: Lésions du genou. J. Radiol. Electrol 40 (1959), 418
–, L. MOLÉ, R. PETER: Apport de la tomographie dans l'étude des lésions du genou par le procédé du double contraste. Note prelim. J. Radiol. Electrol. 41 (1950), 79
FOURNIER, A., G. LAVRANURS, J. RANQUE, G. TRANIER: Incidences de la technique sur les complications possibles de l'arthrographie du genou. J. Radiol. Electrol 41 (1960), 358
FRICK, P.: Neue Röntgenuntersuchungen am Kniegelenk. Fortschr. Röntgenstr. 46 (1932), 155
FUERMAIER, A.: In: Holmann, Hackenbroch und Linemann. Handbuch der Orthopädie. G. Thieme, Stuttgart 1957
FUNKE, T.: Radiography of the knee joint. Med. Radiogr. Photogr. 36 (1960), 1

GALLAND, M.: Un procédé radiographique rélévateur des cartilages et synoviales articulaires. Rev. Orthop. 22 (1935), 743
GASCO PASCUAL, J., J. SALA DE PABLO: L'atrografia de la rodilla para el diagnostico de los traumas meniscales. Rev. Clin. Espan. 2 (1940), 147
GEIST, R. M., C. C. WHITSETT, C. R. HUGHES: Diodrast arthrography of the knee joint. Brit. J. Radiol. 25 (1952), 120
GERTSOVSKII, S. L., M. P. MIKHAGKIN: Kontrastnaia artrografiia pri provrezhdenii meniskov kolennoga sustava. Vest. rentg. 33 (1958), 45
GIACOBBE, G.: Pneumoartro terapeutico nelle lesioni articolari del ginocchio. Arch. ital. Chir. 12 (1927), 433
GIRAUDI, G., R. MERZIANI: Sull'impiego dell'Uroselectan B nello studio roentgenologico delle articolazioni. Atti II Congresso ital. Radiol. med. 2 (1934), 295
–, R. MARZIANI: Nota preventiva sull'impiego dell'Uroselectan B nello studio roentgenologico delle articolazioni. Arch. Ortop. (Milan) 50 (1934), 757
GRADYEVITSCH, B.: Arthrographie dans les maladies du genou. J. belge Radiol. 26 (1937), 333
GROB, H.: Der Meniskusschaden des Kniegelenkes als Unfall- und Aufbrauchsfolge. F. Enke, Stuttgart 1954
GROSSMANN, MINOR: Roentgen demonstration of the semilunar cartilages of the knee. Amer. J. Roentgenol. 53 (1945), 454
GSCHWEND, N.: Die Osteochondritis dissecans tali. Z. Unfallmed. Berufskr. 53 (1960), 293

HÁJEK, V.: Tomoarthrography. Čs. Rentgenol. 12 (1958), 182
HARTUNG, F.: Über Ganglienbildung am medialen Kniegelenksmeniscus. Arch. orthop. Unfall-Chir. 47 (1955), 149
HASEGAWA, K.: Arthrography of meniscal lesions of the knee joint. Nagova J. med. Sci. 22 (1959), 22
Arthrography of meniscal lesions of the knee joint. Nagoya J. med. Sci. 22 (1959), 85
HAUCK, P. P.: Arthrography. I. A comparative study of arthrography of the knee joint. Brit. J. Radiol 25 (1952), 120
HÄUPTLI, O.: Die Pneumoarthrographie des Kniegelenkes. Schweiz. med. Wschr. 77 (1947), 549
HAYK, W.: Frühdiagnose des lateralen Meniscuscystoms. Wien klin. Wschr. 65 (1953), 180
HEER, W.: Zur Technik der Arthro-Pneumographie nach Bircher. Schweiz. med. Wschr. 62 (1932), 429

HEIM, U.: Fehlbefunde am lateralen Meniscus. Helv. Chir. Acta 30 (1963) 110.
HELENON, C., J. LATASTE: L'artrographie du genou. Cah. Coll. Méd. Hôp. Paris 2 (1961), 597
HENRICHSEN, A.: Meniscusverkalkung im Röntgenbild. Röntgenpraxis, 4 (1932), 403
HERZOG, E. G.: Air arthrography in diagnosis of torn semilunar cartilage, Lancet 1945/II, 5
HERZOG, R.: Über Meniskusschäden und Meniskusoperation unter kritischer Würdigung von rund 500 operierten Fällen. Münch. med. Wschr. 95 (1953), 1076
HENSCHEN, C.: Die mechanischen Arbeitsschäden des Kniegelenkes. Schweiz. med. Wschr. 59 (1929), 1368
HILGENREINER, R.: Zur Frage der Kniegelenksmeniscusdarstellung im Röntgenbild. Zbl. Chir. 59 (1932), 7
HOFFA, A.: Über Röntgenbilder nach Einblasung von Sauerstoff in das Kniegelenk, Berl. klin. Wschr. 43 (1906), 28
HOFFMANN, H. G.: Schienbeinkopfbrüche. Zbl. Chir. 68 (1941), 1342
HOLMGREN, B. S.: Flüssiges Fett im Kniegelenk nach Trauma. Acta radiol. 23 (1942), 131
HOOPER, R. S., W. E. SPRING: Popliteal aneurysm after lateral meniscectomy. J. Bone Surg. 35 (1953), 272
HOPF, A.: Die Röntgendarstellung des Kniegelenkes. Z. Otrhop. 80 (1951), 358
HORISBERGER, B.: Über Vorkommen, Entstehung und Behandlung des Meniscusriß. Helv. chir. Acta 26 (1959), 128
HOSFORD, J. P.: Arthrogram to show extent of synovial cavity after synovectomy. Proc. Roy. Soc. Med. 30 (1937), 1264
HUNGER, H.: Kontrastdarstellung des Kniegelenkes in der Diagnostik der Meniskusverletzungen. Mschr. Unfallheilk. 60 (1957), 102
HURTER, E.: Echte Lipome des Meniscus. Arch. orthop. Unfall-Chir. 47 (1955), 399

JAKOBY, E.: Erfahrungen bei Meniscusverletzungen beim Scheibenmeniscus und Meniscusganglion. Arch. orthop. Unfall-Chir. 46 (1954), 290
JEANNOPOULOS, C. L.: Observation on discoid menisci. J. Bone Surg. 32 A (1950), 649
JELINEK, R.: Über Meniscus-, Seitenband- und Kreuzbandverletzungen des Kniegelenkes. Wien. klin. Wschr. 67 (1955), 931
Beitrag zur Diagnose der Meniscusverletzungen. Wien med. Wschr. 69 (1957), 547
JENSEN, S. B., P. TH. ANDERSEN: Arthrography as a diagnostic aid – in lesions of the knee joint. Acta chir. scand. 103 (1952), 302
JEWSTROPOW, A. P., A. E. ABOLINA: Neuartige Kniegelenkeröffnung bei Meniscusriß. Zbl. Chir. 86 (1961), 1027
JONASCH, E.: Zur Klassifizierung der Arthrose im Kniegelenk. Z. Orthop. 91 (1959), 579
Die Erkennung der Interposition eines Knieseitenbandes nach dessen Zerreißung. Fortschr. Röntgenstr. 91 (1959), 403
Über die röntgenologische Schattenbildung an der Innen- und Außenseite des Kniegelenkes. Arch. orthop. Unfall-Chir. 50 (1959), 361
Über das Auftreten von Knochenveränderungen bei Cysten des lateralen Meniscus des Kniegelenkes. Fortschr. Röntgenstr. 93 (1960), 466
JUNGHAGEN, S.: La pneumographie du genou surtout dans les cas de lipoma arborisant. Acta radiol 14 (1933), 172
JÜRGENS, B.: Anwendung von Sauerstoffeinblasung in das Kniegelenk. Zbl. Chir. 56 (1929), 9100

KAARMANN, A.: Die beruflichen Voraussetzungen des Bergmannmeniscus (Berufskrankheit No. 26). Mschr. Unfallheilk. 61 (1958), 39
Die chirurgischen Berufskrankheiten. F. Enke, Stuttgart 1958
KAINBERGER, F.: Ergebnisse der Darstellung des Gelenksraumes insbesondere des Kniegelenkes mit Hilfe der Doppelkontrastmethode. Wien klin. Wschr. 73 (1961), 302
KARCHER, H.: Der Wert der Kniegelenkdarstellung mit Uroselectan B. Chirurg 12 (1940), 734
KEBEKUS, H.: Die Bedeutung der Arthrographie für die Diagnostik der Kniebinnenschäden. Knappschaftsarzt 25 (1960), 197

KELLER, H.: Estudios experimentales en la visualizacion de la rodilla mediante contraste. Proc. Soc. ecp. Med. Biol. 27 (1930), 85
Series artograficas como medio de diagnostico. Intern J. Med. 78 (1931), 44
KESSLER, J., Z. SILVERMAN, F. NISSIM: Arthrography of the knee. A critical study of errors and their sources. Amer. J. Roentgenol. 86 (1961), 359
–, Z. SILVERMAN, F. NISSIM: Diagnosis of lesions of the posterior horn of the medial meniscus. Harefuah 59 (1960), 269
KLAMI, P., M. KURKIPÄÄ: Tomoarthrography of meniscal lesions of the knee-joint; fifteen verified cases. Acta radiol. (Stockh.), 48, (1957), 248
KLEINBERG, S.: Die diagnostische Sauerstofffüllung der Gelenke. Amer. J. Surg. 35 (1921), 256
Sauerstoffeinblasung in das Gelenk als diagnostisches Hilfsmittel. Arch. Surg. Amer. 8 (1924), 827
Lungenembolie nach Sauerstoffeinblasung ins Knie J. A. M. A. 89 (1929), 172
KNOLL, MATTHIES: Darstellung von Gelenken mittels Jodipin-Einfüllung. Fortschr. Röntgenstr. 43 (1931), 1
KÖHLER, A., E. A. ZIMMER: Borderlands of the Normal and Early Pathologic in Skeletal Roentgenology. 3rd ed. translated by S. Wilk. Grune & Stratton, New York and London, 1969
KÖRBEL, K.: Beitrag zur Morphologie und Behandlung der Gelenkchondromatose. Chirurg 32 (1961), 473
KÖSTLER, J.: Die Blutgefäßversorgung der Menisken und ihre Bedeutung bei der Heilung von Meniskusrissen. Arch. klin. Chir. 187 (1936), 15
KREUSCHER, PH., H. KELIKIAN: The use of iodized oil (lipiodol and jodipin) in the diagnosis of joint lesions. Surgery 50 (1930), 888
KROEMER, K.: Der verletzte Meniscus, 3rd ed. W. Maudrich, Vienna–Bonn 1955
Die röntgenologische Darstellung des Kniegelenk-Innenraumes durch Kontrastfüllung und die Deutung der Befunde. Chirurg 9 (1937), 449
Über die Radiographie der Gelenke. Klin. Med. 2 (1947), 29

LACHOWIEZ, A., M. M. GOLDMANN: Die Pneumoradiographie in der Diagnostik der Kniegelenkerkrankungen. Pol. Przegl. radiol. 10/11 (1936), 35
LANG, F.: Meniscushistologie und unfallmedizinische Beurteilung der Zwischenknorpelläsionen. Z. Unfallmed. Berufskr. 39 (1946), 177
LARGARDE, C., R. RAVELEAU, M. LE GUIFFANT, E. ESQUIROL, E. LAURENS: Six ans de pratique de l'arthrographie opaque du genou. (Analyse d'une série personelle de 567 examens). J. Radiol. Électrol 41 (1960), 353
LEROUX, G., J. M. COLLETTE: Arthrographie opaque et mixte simultanée du genou. Etude comparative des images. J. Radiol. Électrol. 41 (1960), 355
LEWIN, P.: The Knee and Related Structures. Lea & Febiger, Philadelphia 1952
LI CASTRI PATTI, L., G. SALOMONE: L'artografia del ginocchio cor doppio mezzo di contrasto. Sicilia sanit. 12 (1959), 153
LICOPPE, G.: Mixed iodo-air arthrography-Routine examination in the diagnosis of internal lesions of the knee. Acta belg. Arte med. pharm. milit. 112 (1959), 288
LINDBLOM, K.: Arthrography of the knee joint. Acta radiol. (Stockh.), Suppl. VII, 1948
LINDE, G.: Unfallzusammenhang bei Meniscusverletzungen der Bergleute. Mschr. Unfallheilk. 31 (1930), 60
LIDSTRÖM, A.: Trauma and ganglia of the semilunar cartilages of the knee, Acta orthop. scand. 23 (1954), 237
LÖWE, J.: Beitrag zur Diagnostik der Meniscusverletzungen des Kniegelenkes unter besonderer Berücksichtigung des Rauberschen Röntgenzeichens. Zbl. Chir. 87 (1962), 721
LONG, L.: Non-injection method for roentgenographic visualization of the internal semilunar cartilage. Amer. J. Roentgenol. 52 (1944), 269

MACH, F.: Arthography of the knee, with a combined injection. Čas, Lék, čes. 96 (1957), 554
MAGNUSSON, W.: Über die Bedingungen des Hervortretens der wirklichen Gelenkspalte auf dem Röntgenbilde. Acta radicl. (Stockh.) 18 (1937), 733

MAGNUS, G.: Unsere Stellung in der Meniscusfrage. Zbl. Chir. 65 (1938), 2380
MANDL, F.: Rearthrotomie – nach Meniscusoperation. Zbl. Chir. 79 (1954), 1169
Beobachtungen und Ergebnisse bei 400 Meniskusoperationen. Dtsch. Z. Chir. 239 (1933), 580
Weitere Beobachtungen zur Regeneration des Meniskus. Zbl. Chir. 62 (1935), 1778
MANFREDI, F.: La stratigrafia nel pneumoartro del ginocchio. Quad. Radiol. 15 (1952), 207
MARTIN, C. G., A. C. CONNOR: Diagnosis of torn meniscus. Amer, J. Surg. 102 (1961), 573
MAU, H.: Die Osteochondritis dissecans und freie Körper des Sprunggelenkes. Z. Orthop. 91 (1959), 582
MCGAW, W. H., E. C. WECKENSER: Arthropneumography of the knee. J. Bone Jt. Surg. 27 (1945), 452
MCMURRAY, T. P.: The semilunar cartilages. Brit. J. Surg. 29 (1942), 407
MERKE, F.: Richtlinien zur Diagnose der Meniscusverletzung. Schweiz. med. Wschr. 70 (1940), 715
MERLE D'AUBIGNÉ, SERRA DE OLIVEIRA, POLONY, CASTAING: Arthrographie du genou pour lésions méniscales (39 cas) Mém. Acad. Chir. 14 (1953), 58
MEYER, P.: Medizinischer Leitfaden zur privaten Unfall- und Haftpflichtversicherung. H. Huber, Berne–Stuttgart 1958
MICHAELIS, L.: Über eine neue Art der Kontrastfüllung des Kniegelenkes. Arch. klin. Chir. 162 (1930), 128
MIESCHAN, I., W. H. MCGAW: Newer methods of pneumoarthrography of the knee-joint with an evaluation of the procedure in 315 observed cases. Radiology 49 (1947), 675
MOEHLMANN, MADLENER: Zur Kontrastdarstellung des Kniegelenkes. Fortschr. Röntgenstr. 65 (1942), 51
MOMMSEN, F.: Eine neue horizontale Schnittführung für Eingriffe am inneren Meniscus (insbes. Hinterhorn). Zbl. Chir. 78 (1953), 150
MOREL, J., P. BASTIEN, VANVELCERRABER: La régénération des ménisques du genou après méniscectomie. Rev. Chir. orthopéd. 38 (1952), 137
MUCCHI, L.: L'artrografia del ginocchio con mezzi di contrasto transparenti ed opachi. Atti Soc. lombard. chir. 5 (1957), 14
MÜLLER, LAUBER: Experimentelle Untersuchungen über die Gelenkresorption unter verschiedenen physikalischen Bedingungen. Bruns' Beitr. klin. Chir. 155 (1932), 39
MURDOCH, G.: Congenital discoid medial semilunar cartilage. J. Bone Jt. Surg. 38 (1956), 564
MURRAY, R. C., E. FORRAI: Transitory eosinophilia localised in the knee joint after pneumoarthrography. J. Bone Jt. Surg. 32 (1950), 74

NAGURA, S.: Zur Aetiologie der Coxa vara, zugleich ein Beitrag zur Kenntnis der Transformation des Knochens. Arch. klin. Chir. 199 (1940), 533
NAGY, J., F. POLGAR: Beiträge zur Röntgenanatomie des kontrastgefüllten Kniegelenkes. Fortschr. Röntgenstr. 45 (1932), 688
NATALE, L.: Le lesioni traumatiche dei menischi. Sintomatologia, diagnosi, terapia e risultati. Atti Soc. Lombard. Chir. 3 (1935), 1461
NIDECKER, H. H.: Die gezielte Pneumoarthrographie des Kniegelenkes. Radiol. clin. (Basle) 22 (1953), 10
NICOLET, A.: La pathogénie et le traitment des lésions du ménisque. Acta orthop. belg. 19 (1953), 281
NOIX, M.: Etude radiocinématographique des ménisques du genou. J. de Radiol. 38 (1957), 531
NORDHEIM, G.: Eine neue Methode, den Gelenkknorpel, besonders die Kniegelenkmeniskem, röntgenologisch darzustellen. Fortschr. Röntgenstr. 57 (1938), 479
NOVOLODSKII, L. P.: Rentgenologicheskie simptomy povrezhdeniia meniskov kolennogo sustava pri kontrastnoi artrografii. Vestn. Rentgenol. Radiol 34 (1959), 71

OBERHOLZER, J.: Die Pneumoarthrographie. Beitr. klin. Chr. 158 (1933), 112
Die Technik der Pneumoradiographie des Kniegelenkes nach Bircher. Zbl. Chir. 60 (1933), 1522
Einige ausgewählte Pneumoradiographiebilder des Kniegelenkes. Röntgenpraxis 6 (1934), 646

L'arthro-pneumoradiographie (méthode de Bircher). J. Radiol. Électrol. 20 (1936), 18
Ergänzung zur Technik der Pneumoradiographie der Gelenke und besonders des Kniegelenkes. Zbl. Chir. 63 (1936), 2117
Röntgendiagnostik der Gelenke mittels der Doppelkontrastmethode. G. Thieme, Leipzig 1938
OGGIONI, G. L.: L'artrografia del ginocchio nella diagnosi di menisco discale. Arch. Putti Chir. Organi Mov. 1 (1951), 276
L'artrografia del ginocchio nella diagnosi di lesione meniscale. Ann. Radiol. diagn. 21 (1949), 77
DE OLIVEIRA, S.: Ménisque du genou. Etude arthropneumographique de leur régénération après méniscectomie. Rev. Chir. orthop. 40 (1954), 212
OTTONELLO, P.: I movimenti dell'articolazione del ginocchio dal punto di vista radiologico. Nunt. radiol. (Rome) 25 (1959), 691

PACINI, D.: Lesione del menisco ed artrografia. Radioter. Radiobiol. Fis. med. 3 (1936), 159
PERINI, G.: L'artrografia. Radioter. Radiobiol. Fis. med. (1934), 293
PHILIPPON, J.: Etude radiologique des ligaments croisés du genou. J. Radiol. Électrol. 38 (1957), 257
Etude des malformations congénitales méniscales par arthropneumographie. J. Radiol. Électrol. 40 (1959), 1
–, A. EYCHENNE: Le gonarthrographe. J. Radiol. Électrol. 39 (1958), 907

QUANTANCE, P. A.: Pneumoroentgenography of the knee joint. Analysis of fifty cases. J. Bone Jt. Surg. 20 (1938), 353
QUARANTA, M., G. SENIS: L'artrostratigrafia con contrasto opaco nella diagnostica delle lesioni meniscali del ginocchio. Clin. ortop. 8 (1956), 6

RAKOFSKY, M.: Air injection as an aid in the diagnosis of internal derangements of the knee. Amer. J. Med. 63 (1950), 502
RAUBER, A.: Ein wenig bekanntes Röntgensymptom bei alten Meniscusaffektionen. Z. Unfallmed. Berufskr. 37 (1944), 168
Schließt ein negativer Operationsbefund eine Meniscusverletzung aus? Praxis 46 (1957), 734
RAUENBUSCH, L.: Zur Röntgendiagnostik der Meniskusverletzungen des Kniegelenkes. Fortschr. Röntgenstr. 10 (1906), 350
RECHTMANN, A. M.: Pneumarthrosis of the knee. Surg. Gynec. Obstet. 49 (1929), 683
REDINI, G.: Contributo allo studio delle cisti del menisco. Minerva ortop. (Turin) 7 (1956), 403
Il menisco discoide. Clin. ortop. 5 (1953), 225
REHBEIN, F.: Die Entstehung der Osteochondritis dissecans. Dtsch. Z. Chir. 265 (1950), 69
REMEN, D.: Beitrag zur Diagnose und Therapie des Meniscusschadens unter besonderer Berücksichtigung der Doppelkontrastarthrographie. Diss. Zürich 1961.
REZEK, J.: Die Arthrographie. Fortschr. Röntgenstr. 89 (1958), 319
RIEUNAU, J., P. FICAT, R. RIVIERE: Arthrographie opaque et lésions traumatiques du genou. Acta orthop. belg. 20 (1954), 421
RITTER, U.: Zur Klinik und Röntgendiagnose der Meniscusverkalkungen. Chirurg 23 (1952), 22
RITZMANN, K. M.: Ergebnisse der Behandlung von Meniscusschäden in den Jahren 1936–1945. Diss. Zürich 1951
ROCZEN, J.: Zwei bemerkenswerte Fälle von Meniscusläsionen und ihre röntgenologische Erfassung durch Kontrastfüllung Zbl. Chir. 64 (1937), 629
ROLLO, S.: L'impiego dei mezzi di contrasto nell'esame radiografico dell'articolazione del ginocchio, con speciale riguardo allo studio delle lesioni dei menischi. Chir. Organi Mov. 20 (1934), 463
ROSEN, J. E.: Unusual intrameniscal lunulae. Tress case reports. J. Bone Jt. Surg. 40 (1958), 925
ROYER, M.: Arthrographie du genou. Laval. méd. 31 (1961), 57
RUTISHAUSER, E., G. MAJUO: Les lésions osseuses par surcharge dans le squelette normal. Schweiz. med. Wschr. 79 (1949), 281
RUTSCHEIDT, F.: Pneumoradiographische Nachuntersuchungen über Meniscusersatzgewebe. Z. Orthop. 88 (1956), 179
RÜTTIMANN, A.: Die Doppelkontrastarthrographie des Kniegelenkes. Fortschr. Röntgenstr. 87 (1957), 736

–, M. DEL BUONO: Was leistet die Doppelkontrastarthrographie in der Kniegelenkdiagnostik. Chir. Praxis 1 (1959), 107

SACHS, M. D., W. H. McGAW, P. RUSSEL, M. D. RIZZO: Studies in the scope of pneumoarthrography of the knee as a diagnostic aid. Radiology 54 (1950), 11
SALOTTI, A.: Sulla visibilità dei menischi del ginocchio. Nunt. radiol (Rome) 10 (1942), 309
SAVITSKY, Y. N., G. N. TREISTER: Contrast tomography of the knee joint in injury of meniscus. Vestn. Rentgenol. Radiol. 34 (1959), 40
SCHAEFER, H. G.: Zur Rearthrotomie des Kniegelenkes, zugleich ein Beitrag zur Regeneration des Meniscus. Zbl. Chir. 78 (1953), 1048
SCHAER, H.: Der Meniscusschaden. G. Thieme, Leipzig 1938
SCHAERER, K.: Die Arthrographie des Kniegelenkes mit positivem Kontrastmittel. Radiol. clin. (Basle) 22 (1953), 528
SCHARIGER, E.: Fehler bei der Diagnose von Meniscusverletzung. Mschr. Unfallheilk. 60 (1957), 4
SCHILLING, H.: Vollständige oder teilweise Meniscusentfernung? Mschr. Unfallheilk. 66 (1963), 82
SCHLÄFLI, O.: Die Erfahrungen der Anstalt auf dem Gebiete der Meniscusschäden in den letzten 10 Jahren. Z. Unfallmed. Berufskr. 37 (1944), 223
SCHLÜTER, K., R. BECKER: Fehlform des äußeren Meniscus als Ursache des schnappenden Kniegelenkes. Chirurg 25 (1954), 499
–, R. BECKER, W. BERCHTOLD: Zur Aetiologie und Pathogenese der endoartikulären Myxofibrose des Kniegelenkes, sog. Meniscuscysten. Chirurg 27 (1956), 343
SCHNAUDER, A.: Die Meniscusdegeneration und ihre Deutung im Doppelkontrastarthrogramm. Fortschr. Röntgenstr. 96 (1962), 120
SCHNEIDER, P.G.: Die Technik der lateralen Meniscektomie. Chirurg 33 (1962), 311
SCHOEN, H.: Zur Technik der Gelenk-Kontrast-Darstellung. Röntgenpraxis 12 (1940), 363
SCHROP, F. J.: Zur Genese der primären Meniscusverkalkungen. Fortschr. Röntgenstr. 76 (1952), 202
SCHÜLLER, J.: Der Wert der Röntgenkontrastdarstellung des Kniegelenkes. Röntgenpraxis 4 (1932), 947
Die Kontrastdarstellung der Gelenke. Z. Orthop. 64 (1936), 318
SCHUM, H.: Das Pneumoradiogramm des Kniegelenkes. Dtsch. Z. Chir. 1/2, (1932), 947
Die Pneumoradiographie des Kniegelenkes und ihre praktischen Ergebnisse. Dtsch. med. Wschr. 58 (1933), 1659
SENN, H.: Zur Behandlung der Tibiakopffrakturen. Diss. Zurich 1961
SERRA DE OLIVEIRA: Arthropneumographie pour lésions méniscales. Rev. Chir. orthop. 40 (1954), 32
SEYSS, R.: Arthrographie des Kniegelenkes. Technik, Erfahrungen, Ergebnisse und Indikation. Arch. orthop. Unfall-Chir. 48 (1956), 403
SHAPIRO: Wann man einen Kniegelenkmeniskus im Röntgenbild zu sehen bekommt. Zbl. Chir. 23 (1929),
SIEVERS, R.: Röntgenographie der Gelenke mit Jodipin. Fortschr. Röntgenstr. 35 (1928), 16
SIMON, H.T., A. S. HAMILTON, C. L. FARRINGTON: Pneumography of the knee; A newer technic demonstrating its value in the diagnosis of semilunar cartilage injury. J. Bone Jt. Surg. 28 (1946), 540
SLANY, A.: Autoptische Reihenuntersuchungen an Kniegelenken mit besonderer Berücksichtigung der Meniskuspathologie. Arch. Orthop. 41 (1941), 256
SMILIE, J.S.: The congenital discoid meniscus. J. Bone Jt. Surg. 30 (1948), 671
Injuries of the Knee Joint. 2nd ed. Livingstone, Edinburgh 1951
Osteochondritis dissecans. Livingstone, Edinburgh & London 1960
Observations on the regeneration of the semilunar cartilages in man. Brit. J. Surg. 31 (1944), 298
Injures of the Knee Joint. Livingstone, Edinburgh 1946
SMITH, F.B., H.C. BLAIR: Tibial collateral ligament strain due to occult derangements of the medial meniscus. J. Bone Jt. Surg. 36 (1954), 88

SODDEMANN, H.: Die Begutachtung von Meniscusschäden bei Bergleuten, die außerdem regelmäßig Sport betrieben haben. Mschr. Unfallheilk. 66 (1963), 21

SOMERVILLE, E. W.: Air arthrography as an aid in diagnosis of lesions of the menisci of the knee joint. J. Bone Jt. Surg. 28 (1946), 451

SPIRA, E.: Über die Diagnose und Behandlungserfolge bei Verletzungen der Menisken. Beitr. klin. Chir. 158 (1933), 157

SPRINGORUM, P. W.: Wandel der Anamnese bei Meniscusschäden. Mschr. Unfallheilk. 62 (1959), 8
Meniscuslaesion bei Jugendlichen. Zbl. Chir. 84 (1959), 1581
Die Formen des Meniscusrisses. Mschr. Unfallheilk. 65 (1962), 311
Alter und Meniscusschaden. Mschr. Unfallheilk. 65 (1962), 464

STARK, W.: Zur Wahl des Verfahrens bei der Kniegelenks-Kontrastdarstellung. Zbl. Chir. 68 (1941), 445
Erfahrungen mit der Röntgenkontrastdarstellung des Kniegelenkes. Ed. Barth. Leipzig 1942

STÖR, O.: Die Röntgendarstellung der inneren Kniegelenkverletzungen nach Böhm. Arch. klin. Chir. 177 (1933), 171
Röntgenologische Gelenkdarstellung. Münch. med. Wschr. 77 (1935), 1075

STOCKER, H.: Zur Darstellung der Meniski und Kreuzbänder durch die Arthrographie mit Uroselectan B. Dtsch. Z. Chir. 11/12 (1935), 445

STRATA, A.: Un nuovo caso di meniscite del ginocchio. Minerva ortop. (Turin) 4 (1953), 418

STRELI, R.: Meniscotom für die partielle Meniscusresektion. Chirurg. 27 (1956), 94
Über eine Meniscussonde. Chirurg. 27 (1956), 75
Spätergebnisse nach partieller Meniscectomie bei 82 Fällen. Chirurg. 26 (1955), 97

STUMPFEGGER, L.: Meniscusvernarbung nach Schienbeinkopfbrüchen. Arch. klin. Chir. 189 (1937), 226

TERRACOL, J., L. J. COLANERI: Meniskusverletzungen und Luftaufblähung des Gelenkes. Presse méd. 29 (1921), 113

TESCHENDORF, W.: Zur Verwendung eines leicht resorbierbaren Gases (Stickoxydul) für die Darstellung der Gelenke und des Pneumoperitoneums. Fortschr. Röntgenstr. 53 (1936), 476

TOBLER, TH.: Makroskopische und histologische Befunde am Kniegelenkmeniscus in verschiedenen Lebensaltern. Schweiz. med. Wschr. 56 (1929), 1359

TOLDT, C., F. HOCHSTETTER: Anatomischer Atlas, Vol. I. Urban & Schwarzenberg, Vienna 1947

TREMAGLIA, M.: La pneumoartrografia del ginocchio con Joduron. Minerva ortop. 2/4 (1951), 321

TRENTA, A., C. FIOCCHI: Contributo allo studio della formazione del gas articolare nel ginocchio. Radiologia (Rome) 14 (1958), 1385

TURCO, B.: Il valore del pneumoartro come mezzo diagnostico nelle lesioni dei menischi. Diario Radiol. 5 (1930),

TURNHEER, F.: Die Meniscusrisse des Jahres 1945 im Krankengut der SUVA. Diss. Zurich 1947

TURNER, V. C., F. B. WURTZ: Arthrography in the diagnosis of meniscal injuries of the knee. J. Bone Jt. Surg. 41 (1959), 1213

ULRICHS, B.: Röntgenogramme des Kniegelenkes mit Sauerstoffeinblasung. Fortschr. Röntgenstr. 21 (1914), 618
Technik und Ergebnisse der Sauerstoffüllung des Kniegelenkes. Fortschr. Röntgenstr. 43 (1931), 53

UTHGENANNT, H.: Über Nutzen und Nachteil der Arthrographie des Kniegelenkes. Bruns' Beitr. klin. Chir. 188 (1954), 328

VALLS: Lesiones traumaticas de los meniscos, ligamentos cruzados, y ligamentos laterales de la rodilla. Ed. El Ateneo, Buones Aires 1941

VAN CAUWENBERGHE, R., X. Denis: Arthrographie du genou et lésions méniscales traumatiques. Rev. méd. Liège, 16 (1961), 421

VAN DE BERGH, F., M. CREVECOEUR: La méniscographie en série du genou. J. belge Radiol. 34 (1951), 7
–, M. CREVECOEUR: La méniscographie en série du genou. Acta orthop. belg. 19 (1953), 293
–, M. CREVECOEUR: La méniscographie en série du genou (après 1000 examens). J. Radiol. Électrol. 36 (1955), 389

VANDENDORP, F.: La pneumoarthrographie dans les lésions méniscales du genou. J. Radiol. Électrol. 34 (1953), 186

VANDENDORP, F., R. DU BOIS: L'Arthrographie gazeuse dans les lésions méniscales du genou. J. Radiol. Électrol. 41 (1960), 351

VESPIGNANI, L., G. ZORAT: Diagnosi artrografica del menisco discoide. Radiol. med. (Turin) 47 (1961), 208

VILLIERS, A.: Sériographie pour pneumarthrographie du genou. J. de Radiol. 38 (1957), 1085

VITINGOU, J. A.: Znachenie artropnermografii u diagnostike povrezhdenii mrnidkob kolennogo sustava. Vestn. Rentgenol. Radiol. 33 (1958), 49

VUILLEUMIER, C.: Über Meniscuslaesionen. Schweiz. med. Wschr. 93 (1963), 221

WADI, H.: Über die Anwendung eines einfachen Gerätes bei der Kniegelenksarthrographie. Fortschr. Röntgenstr. 95 (1961), 407

WAGNER, W.: Das Sudeck-Syndrom. W. Maudrich, Vienna 1960

WEISMAN, J.: An improved technic for the roentgen demonstrations of the semilunar cartilages of the knee. Amer, J. Med. 63 (1950), 502

WELLER, S., E. KÖHNLEIN: Die Traumatologie des Kniegelenkes. Diagnostik und Therapie. G. Thieme, Stuttgart 1962

WERNDORFF, K. R., H. ROBINSON: Verhandlung d. deutsch. Gesellsch. f. orthop. Chir., 4th Congress, 1905

WIESER, C., U. HEIM: Zur Röntgenanatomie des lateralen Hinterhornes im Kniearthrogramm. Radiol. clin. (Basle) 31 (1962), 264

WITTMOSER, R.: Über die Kniegelenkmeniskushistologie in den ersten zwei Lebensjahrzehnten. Arch. Orthop. 39 (1939), 96

WOLLENBERG, G. A.: Apparat zur Einblasung chemisch reinen Sauerstoffes in die Körpergewebe und in die Körperhöhlen. Med. Klin. 2 (1906), 20
Die normale Anatomie des Kniegelenkes im Röntgenbild nach Aufblasung der Gelenkkapsel. Z. orthop. Chir. 19 (1908), 245

ZAKRISSON, U.: Meniscography with double contrast injection by van de Bergh's method. Nord. Med. 51 (1959), 636

ZELLWEGER, H., M. EBNÖTHER: Helv. paediat. Acta 6 (1951), 95

ZUCCO, C. M.: Articolazioni e lesioni articolari studiate mediante il pneumoartro. Rass. intern. Clin. (1924), 437

ZÜRCHER, W. O.: Die Arthrographie des Kniegelenkes mit positivem Kontrastmittel. Dissertation, Zurich 1953

# Index

Age of meniscus lesion, determination of, 57
Anatomy of the knee joint, 2–6
Apley test, 22–23, 95
Arthritic changes, 23, 98–99, 112, 128
  arthrogram, 99
  differential diagnosis, 98–99
  secondary, 23, 99
Arthrogram
  abnormal, 53 ff.
  arthritic symptoms, 99
  bursae, 47–49
    superimposition of, 88
  cruciate ligament, 51–52
  degenerative meniscus changes, 71–73
  diagnosis, 78 ff.
  differential diagnosis, 93 ff.
    cartilage and bone changes, 98 ff
    collateral ligament and capsular damage, 95–96
    ganglia and tumors, 107–110
    synovitis and bursitis, 105, 107
  ganglion, 107–110
    of the capsule, 110
    of the meniscus, 72–73, 107–108
  joint capsule, 45–47
  joint spaces, 45–47
  hiatus popliteus, 45
  Hoffa's disease, 106–107
  Infrapatellar fad pad, 50
    superimposition of, 85–86
  meniscectomy, status after, 77–78
  meniscus injuries, 58 ff.
  normal, 31 ff.
  osteochondritis dissecans, 99–101
  osteochondromatosis, 103–104
  popliteal fissure. See Hiatus popliteus
  popliteus tendon, 45,
    tendon sheath of, 45
  recessus, 31, 35
    superimposition of, 86–87
  synovitis, 105 ff.
Arthrography
  air, 25
  air filling, 24–25
  complications, 90–91
  contrast media, 26
  double contrast, 25 ff.
  evacuation of joint effusion, 27
  equipment, 28
  historical review, 24–25
  indications, 25
  liquid contrast medium, 29
  materials, 25–26
  methodology, 25 ff.
  puncture of the knee joint, 26
  technic, 26 ff.
  technical errors, 31
  x-ray technic, 29–31

Articular surfaces, 52

Ballottement of the patella, 18
Böhler's sign, 21, 94
Bragard's sign, 20
Bucket-handle tear, 8, 14, 16, 112, 121–122
  resection of, 121
Bursa, 47–49
  openings, 49
  pathologic, 49
  popliteal, 5–6, 49
    diseases, 107
  semimembranosogastrocnemica, 6, 40
  suprapatellar, 49
Bursitis, 105 ff.

Calcification, 23
  dorsal fat pad, 23
  infrapatellar fat pad, 23
  meniscus, 23
Capsular space, 45
  inferior, 45
  superior, 45
Capsule lesions, 93 ff.
Cartilage changes, 98 ff.
  arthrosis deformans, 98-99
  differential diagnosis, 98–99
Chondromalacia patellae, 104, 112
Classification of meniscus lesions, 14–16
Clinical examination, 18–20
Collateral ligament lesion, 93–96
Complications of double contrast arthrography, 90–91
Concentric tears, 55–56
Congenital variations, 9
Constitutional variations, 9
Contrast media, 26
  injection, 27–28
    periarticular, 82–85
Cruciate ligaments, anatomy 5
  arthrogram, 50–51
  lesions of, 96–98
    drawer sign, 5, 19, 98
    recognition in arthrogram, 98

Degenerative changes of the meniscus, 10, 14, 71
Differential diagnosis, 93 ff.
  arthrosis deformans, 98–99
  bursitis, 105–107
  capsule lesions, 93–96
  cartilage and bone changes, 98–105
    osteochondritis dissecans, 99–101
    osteochondromatosis, 103–104
  chondromalacia patellae, 104
  clinical and radiologic, 93 ff.
  collateral ligament lesions, 95–96
    sprains, 94
    tears, 94

Differential diagnosis (*cont.*)
  cruciate ligament lesions, 96–98
  ligamentous and capsule damage, 93–98
    in arthrogram, 95–96
  synovitis, 105–107
Disinsertion, 57
Double contrast arthography
  indications for, 25
Drawer sign, 5, 19, 98
  demonstration of, 19

Errors of diagnosis in arthrogram, 78–89
  of anatomical differentiation, 85–89
Errors, technical, in arthrography, 31
Extension limitation of, 19

False diagnoses, characteristic, in arthrogram, 89
Fat pads, dorsal, 5. 50
  infrapatellar, 5, 50
    calcification of, 23
    hemorrhages in, 50
Forms of tear of the meniscus, 7–8, 13–14, 53 ff.
Flattening of meniscus, 71–72
Fractures, intra-articular, 23
  Holmgren method, 23
  tibial plateau, 12–13
Fragmentation of meniscus, 69, 71

Ganglia, 107–110
  of the capsule, 110
  meniscus, 10, 23, 107–108
    arthrogram, 72
Gas arthrography, 24
"Giving-way" signs, 17–18, 95, 97, 126, 131

Hauffe baths, 128
Hemarthrosis, 23
Hematoma, 125
Hiatus popliteus, typical appearance of, 45
Histologic examination in disability evaluation, 132
History taking, 16–17, 131
Hoffa's disease, 106–107, 112
  arthrogram, 107
  routine x-ray, 107
Hoffa's fat pad. *See* Fat pads, infrapatellar
Holmgren's method, 23
Holmgren's sign, 24
Horizontal tears, 56, 63
Hypermobile meniscus, 14

Imbibition, 71
Immobilization, postoperative, 122–123
Indications
  for arthrography, 25
  for conservative and operative therapy, 111
Industrial injuries, 12
Infantile discoid meniscus, 75
Infection, postoperative, 124–125
Initial symptoms, 17
Intra-articular structures, visualization of, 31

Joint capsule, 3, 5, 45, 47
  arthrogram of, 47
  ganglia involving, 107
  lesions, 93
Joint effusion, 17, 18–19, 131
  demonstration of, 18
  incomplete evacuation of, 85
Joint puncture, 26, 112, 123, 124
Joint space, 5, 45–47
  anterior, 5
  arthrogram, 45
  central, 47
  posterior, 45–47

Knee joint anatomy, 2 ff.
  clinical examination, 18–20
  effusion, 17, 18, 131
  locking, 113–114
  mechanics of movement, 6–7
  puncture, 26, 112, 123, 125
  tumors, 110
  vascular supply, 4–5
  x-ray examination, 23 ff.

Late changes, 15, 112, 130–131
  after ligamentous damage, 15
  after traumatic tear, 15, 111–112, 130–131
*Laxité du ménisque,* 87
Ligamentous damage, 9–10
Locking of the knee, 17–18, 113
Longitudinal tears of the meniscus, 8, 14, 29, 55

McMurray test, 22
Mechanical causes of meniscus lesions, 7–8
Mechanics of movement of the knee joint, 6–7
Mechanism of meniscus injury, 8, 10 ff.
Meniscectomy, 75 ff.
  remnant after, 75–76
  status after, 75–78
"Meniscitis", 14
Meniscopathy, 14, 129
Meniscotomes, description of, 116–117
Meniscus
  anatomy, 3 ff.
  calcification, 23
  connection with the capsule, 3, 89
  cross-section, 35–36
  degenerative changes, 10, 71–73, 129
  developmental anomalies, 75
  disability evalution, 129 ff.
  displacement, 6
  fragmentation, 69, 71
  histopathologic finding, 130–131
  importance of, 110–111
  injury. *See* Meniscus injuries
  lateral, 4
    visualization of, 30
  longitudinal tears, 8, 14, 29, 55
  medial, 3
    visualization of, 29–30

Meniscus (*cont.*)
    multiple views, 30–31
        variations in medial, 36–41
    normal, in arthrogram, 31–45
        variations in lateral, 44–45
    recessus, 31, 35, 38–39, 44, 45
    transverse tears, 8, 14, 29, 56–57
    variations in, 36–45
    variations in form, 9
    visualization of, 28 ff.
    x-ray technic, 29–31
Meniscus ganglia, 10, 23, 72, 107–110
    resection of, 122
Meniscus injuries, 53–71, 129
    age of, 57
    complicated tear forms, 59–64
    destruction, 70
    defects, 66–69
    disinsertion, 55
    frequency, 7, 54
    horizontal tear, 56–63
    vertical tear, 54, 55, 61
    with tibial plateau fracture, 12–13
Meniscus lesion
    classification of, 14–16
    disability evaluation, 129 ff.
    pathogenesis, 7 ff.
Meniscus signs, 20–23
*Ménisque allongé,* 87
*Ménisque en virgule inversée,* 75
Merke's sign, 21
Multiple views, 30–31, 52–53

Neuroma formation, 125

Oblique tears, 10, 55–56
Operative treatment, 114 ff.
    anesthesia, 117
    after-care, 112–124
    difficulties, 122
    incision, 118–120
    indications for, 111–112
    instruments, 116–117
    partial or total resection, 114–116
    positioning and tourniquet control, 118
    postoperative complications, 124–128
    preparation, 117
    technic of resection, 114, 120–122
Osteochondritis dissecans, 99, 101, 112
    arthrogram, 101
    x-ray, 101
Osteochondromatosis, 103–104
    arthrogram, 103, 104
    diagnosis, 104
    x-ray, 104

Pain, postoperative, 124
    indicating Sudeck's dystrophy, 127
Partial discoid meniscus, 75
Patella, ballottement of, 18

Pathogenesis
    congenital variations of form, 9
    constitutional factors, 9
    degenerative changes, 10
    fractures of the tibial plateau, 12–13
    industrial injuries, 12
    ligamentous damage, 9–10
    mechanical causes, 7–8
    sports injury, 11–12
    work activies, 12
Payr's sign, 21
Pellegrini-Stieda shadow, 23, 95
Periarticular air injection, excessive, 31
Plaster immobilization, 113
Plica synovialis infrapatellaris, 50
Popliteal artery, injury when resecting meniscus, 122
Popliteal fissure. *See* Hiatus popliteus; Popliteus
    tendon sheath
Popliteus tendon, 45
    sheath, 45
Postmeniscectomy complaints, 78
Postoperative complications, 124–128
    arthrosis deformans, 128
    chronic synovitis, 126–127
    disturbances of wound healing, 125
    infection, 124–125
    meniscus remnants, 126
    pain, 124
    quadriceps weakness, 126
    Sudeck's dystrophy, 127–128
Pseudo-primary degeneration, 15, 16

Quadriceps atrophy, 18, 114, 126, 131
Quadriceps training, 113, 123, 126

Radiation exposure, 93
Ratio of medial to lateral meniscus lesions, 7
Rauber's sign, 23
Recessus, 31, 35
    superior, 49
Reduction of dislocated meniscus, 113
Resection technic, 114, 120–122
Ring-shaped meniscus, 75

Seroma, subcutaneous, 125
Snapping knee, 23
Spontaneous detachment of the meniscus, 15, 112
Sports injuries, 7, 9, 11–12, 131
Sprain *vs.* meniscus lesion, 94
Steinmann's sign
    first, 21
    second, 20
Sudeck's dystrophy, 127–128
Suture complications, 125
Swinging injury, 12
Synovitis, 105–107, 126–127
    chronic, 105–106, 126–127
        arthrogram, 105–106
    villous, 23, 107
        arthrogram, 107

routine x-ray, 107
Tears, fresh traumatic, 15, 111
Tenderness, as diagnostic sign, 19
Therapeutic problems, 110–128
Thickening of meniscus, 72
Tibial plateau fracture and meniscus injury, 12–13, 111
Tomography, 31
Tongue-shaped tear, 13, 14, 21
Transverse tears of the meniscus, 8, 10, 14, 29, 56–57
Traumatic tears
    fresh, 111
    late changes following, 15, 111–112, 130–131
Treatment
    conservative, 112–114
    operative, 114–123
Treatment, principles of, 110–111
Tumors of the knee joint, 110
Typical lesions, 13–14

Unna's paste boot, 113

Vascular supply to the knee joint, 4–5
Vastus medialis, atrophy of, 18
Vulnerability, factors increasing, 9–13

Wound healing, disturbances of, 125

X-ray examination, 23 ff., 95
    calcification of the dorsal fat pad, 23
    capsular ganglion, 109
    chondromalacia patellae, 104
    cruciate ligament lesions, 23, 98
    erosions of bone, 23
    hemarthrosis, 23
    Hoffa's disease, 107
    indications for, 23
    intra-articular effusions, 23
    meniscus calcification, 24
    osteochondromatosis, 103–104
    osteochondritis dissecans, 101
    tumors of the knee joint, 110
X-ray technic, 29–31
    errors in, 85